MTHFR

Whole Food Cookbook & Meal Plans

(The 85% Solution Cook Book)

By Dan Purser MD

Introduction

I want to thank you and congratulate you for downloading the book, **"MTHFR, Whole Food Cookbook and Meal Plans."**

Do you suffer from inexplicable bouts of fatigue or exhaustion during the day? Do you have chronic pain or ailments that don't seem to have a single source or cure? Do you feel depressed most days, and don't understand why?

You may be suffering from **MTHFR mutation**.

MTHFR or *MethyleneTetraHydroFolate Reductase* mutation is a condition wherein the body fails to produce the MTHFR enzyme – and without appropriate amounts of this methylation enzyme you cannot appropriately convert sugar (which we humans cannot directly use) to ATP (energy coinage of our bodies) – *this means you're tired all the time.* In ideal condition, this enzyme effectively breaks down folic acid in food and drinks you consume. It utilizes essential amino acids for processing proteins during digestions, for effectively dispensing calories to/from the adipose tissues, and for absorption of antioxidants in the cells.

A **MTHFR mutation** compromises your:

- **Digestive system**, which "hoards" calories into your fat cells instead of converting these into energy you can burn (i.e. ATP). This can cause gut and digestive problems with which you've probably struggled your entire adult life and for which you've received all kinds of possible diagnoses (celiac, gluten intolerance, etc.). All this in turn leads to steady weight gain, poor muscle development, and even muscle loss. In extreme cases wherein the body fails to properly metabolize proteins, MTHFR mutation leads to higher susceptibility of brittle bones, bone loss, torn muscles, ligature breakage, etc.

  This is also the reason why your body feels heavy and lethargic most of the time.

- **Immune system**, which causes you to feel inexplicably sick on some days, or makes you suffer chronic episodes of deep tissue pain that are unresponsive to most medications and physical therapies. Having a compromised system also means that your immunity is suppressed, making you more susceptible to infectious diseases.

If you already have diabetes, this means your healing abilities are likewise suspect. MTHFR mutation delays physical healing by 50% to 100%, which is dangerous and potentially life-threatening for most diabetics.

If your immune system is compromised, you increase your chances of becoming a bacterial, fungal or viral host. Not only do you become more susceptible to diseases, but you are likely to pass more virulent strains to other people.

- Cerebral circulatory system, which can delay or prevent breakdown of dopamine and serotonin, both of which are needed for cellular repair and for regulating your feelings of elation. MTHFR mutation may be the leading cause of untraceable depression in many people these days.

  A compromised cerebral circulatory system may also cause: autism or ASD (Autism Spectrum Disorder -- 97% of kids with autism have MTHFR disease), ADHD (Attention Deficit Hyperactivity Disorder,) insulin resistance, IBS (Irritable Bowel Syndrome,) Parkinson's disease, schizophrenia, etc.

  Chronic and long-term poor blood circulation can cause nerve damage (particularly in the extremities,) ED or erectile dysfunction in men, numbness or tingling in fingers and toes, forgetfulness, memory loss, and eventually: permanent tissue damage.

This book contains recipes and meal plans on how encourage your body to gradually, and organically develop healthy levels of MTHFR enzymes, which will promote: better digestion, a stronger immune system, and improved blood circulation.

All recipes in this book are healthy, economical, easy to follow, and more importantly, flavorsome.

Thank you again for downloading or purchasing this book. I hope you enjoy it!

Check Out My Other Books
GreatMedEbooks.com

Want to Connect with Dr. Purser?

For women's information on progesterone, testosterone and more download some awesome FREE reports:

www.drpursergifts4women.com

Sign up TODAY to Get Your FREE Reports!

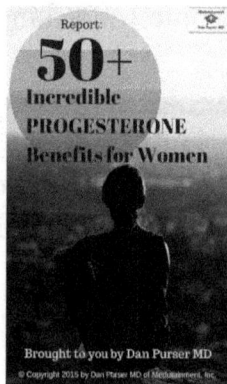

Low levels of progesterone can be treated naturally & optimally in the right situations.

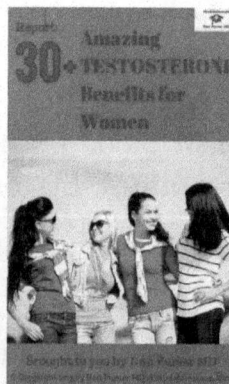

An AMAZING LIST every woman should own – all REFERENCED!

NO FOOLING.

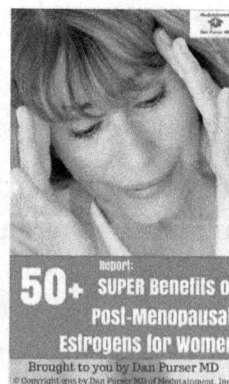

Learn the SUPER BENEFITS of Estrogens in Post-Menopausal Women! This report is fully referenced just for you!

Table of Contents

Chapter 1:   How to Develop MTHFR Meal Plans

The goal for following this diet is to organically increase your body's level of MTHFR enzymes, without using medications or food supplements. Before you start, always consult with your primary health care provider before following a new diet. This is particularly true if you: have any existing medical conditions, are taking powerful medications, and/or are about to (or has recently undergone) surgery of any kind.

To make things easier, remember to create meals that:

1.   Have more whole vegetables in relation to animal protein.

For people with MTHFR mutation, vegetables are easier to digest, as proteins break down longer and are ill-processed by the digestive system. If possible, incorporate larger volume of fresh or lightly cooked vegetables to your meals.

If you prefer having proteins, choose vegetable-based ones (e.g. beans, seeds, nuts, etc.,) or proteins that are less dense in composition, like: eggs, shellfish, or white meat (e.g. fish and poultry.)

2.   Have a little animal protein daily.

This means saying "no" to a strictly vegan diet. A vegan diet needs to be supplemented with Vitamin B12, which is essential for healthy blood and brain functions. Without at least 4 ounces of animal protein per day, the body loses:

- *Creatine,* which is essential for muscle and brain development. It also promotes faster healing.

- *Carnosine,* which delays the body's degenerative processes, and protects against premature aging.

- DHA or *Docosahexaenoic* Acid, or more popularly known as Omega 3 fatty acid, usually found in fish and seafood. Omega 3 can:

- Help lower elevated levels of triglycerides or unwanted fat in the bloodstream. This lessens the risk of all manner of cardiovascular diseases. This also lowers the risk of stroke.
- Promote anti-inflammatory functions. This is a valuable aid when it comes to curbing joint pains and stiffness, especially for people who have or are prone to rheumatoid arthritis. Improved anti-inflammatory functions also help asthmatic people deal with its more painful symptoms.

- Boost levels of dopamine, which can prevent or lessen the onset of depression. It can also ease depressive symptoms of certain mental conditions, like: Alzheimer's disease, bipolar disorder, dementia, and schizophrenia.

3. Have little or no sugar content.

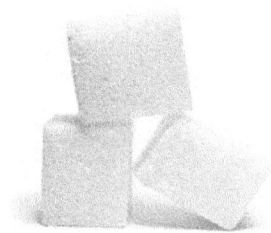

This means lessening your usual consumption of table sugar, and other organic sweeteners. If possible, remove all artificial or man-made sweeteners from your diet. Following a diabetic-friendly diet is advantageous to people who suffer from MTHFR mutation. But if you really must, the only recommended natural sweetener is: ***stevia***.

4. Have starches that are low in the Glycemic Index.

A gluten-free diet is beneficial to people who have Celiac disease, but it can also prove advantageous to people with MTHFR mutation. Subscribing to a gluten-free can ease abdominal muscle cramps, bloating, inexplicable exhaustion or fatigue, intermittent diarrhea, joint pains, mouth sores.

It can also lessen the risk of liver cancer, ease many symptoms of IBS or irritable bowel syndrome, and prevent Dermatitis *herpetiformis*, which is a blistering and itchy skin disease caused by gluten/wheat intolerance.

5. Avoid or severely limit your daily consumption of processed food items and drinks.

Aside from having inordinate levels of salt, sugar and gluten (simple starches or overly processed flour,) these contain man-made additives and preservatives, which can cause all manner of long-term illnesses, particularly diabetes and cancer.

Research also shows a correlation between regular consumption of processed food and the increase of MTHFR mutation incidences.

6. If possible, limit (but do not remove) your daily intake of *methionine*-rich food.

Technically, naturally occurring *methionine* is good for your health. It is an amino acid that breaks down proteins from meals. However, MTHFR diet recommends lessening protein intake. This may inadvertently increase *methionine* level in the bloodstream which can cause: higher levels of acid in urine (which can lead to all manner of urinary tract infections,) and liver damage.

Recommended amount of is only 2 oz. or less per meal. These include: beans, dairy products, meat (beef, eggs, lamb, pork, and turkey,) nuts, seafood, and soy-based products.

7. Limit your daily copper intake (especially if you have high free copper).

Organic copper is essential in the production of blood cells, development of bones, and for the maintenance of brain and heart functions. Again, because you are limiting your animal protein intake, consuming too much copper can lead to all kinds of gastro-intestinal diseases like: abdominal cramps, chronic diarrhea, nausea, and vomiting.

Some food items that contain high levels of copper are (consume sparingly):

- Avocado
- Beans (canned, dried, fresh)
    - Lima beans
    - *Mung* beans
        - Mature beans
        - *Mung* sprouts or sprouted beans
    - Soy beans
- Capers (bottled, canned, fresh)
- Cocoa
    - Breakfast
    - Dry powder, unsweetened
    - Dutch cocoa
- Fermented soy food items and drinks
    - Fermented tofu

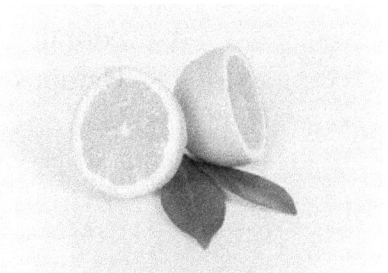

- o *Miso*
- o *Tempeh*
- Goat cheese
- Lemon, raw with zest or peel
- Lentils
- Mushrooms
  - o Brown Italian, raw
  - o *Crimini*, raw
  - o Morel, raw
  - o Portabella, raw
  - o Shiitake mushrooms, cooked
  - o White, cooked
- Nuts
  - o Almonds
  - o Brazil nuts
  - o Cashew nuts
  - o Hazel nuts
  - o Pecan nuts
  - o Pine nuts
  - o Pistachio nuts
  - o Walnuts
- Pulses
  - o Adzuki beans
  - o Kidney beans
  - o Chickpeas or garbanzos
  - o Soy beans
    - ▪ Soy flour
    - ▪ Soy proteins
  - o White beans
- Seafood
  - o Clam (canned or fresh, avoid pickled clams as these contain inordinate amounts of copper)
  - o Crab
  - o Crayfish
  - o Lobster, raw
  - o Mollusks (canned or fresh, avoid pickled mollusk meat as these contain inordinate amounts of copper)
  - o Octopus

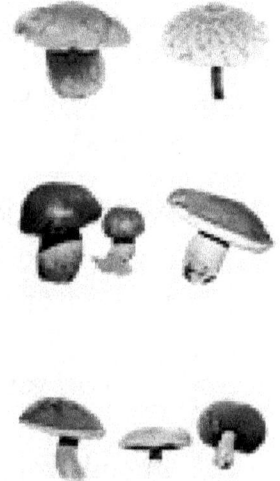

- o Oysters (canned or fresh, avoid pickled oysters as these contain inordinate amounts of copper)
- o Seaweed and/or laver
- o Squid
- o Whelk
  - Seeds
- o Flaxseeds
- o Pumpkin seeds
- o Sesame seeds
  - Dried sesame seeds
- o Sesame butter
- o Sesame paste / tahini
- o Squash
- o Sunflower seeds
- o Watermelon seeds
- Vegetables
  - o Amaranth leaves, cooked or raw
  - o Asparagus, raw
  - o Bamboo shoots, cooked or raw
  - o Basil, fresh (herb)
  - o Beet greens, raw
  - o Fiddlehead ferns, raw
  - o Kale
  - o Napa cabbage, raw
  - o Peppers, fresh
    - *Aji* peppers
    - Banana peppers
    - Bell peppers
    - Bird's eye chilies
    - Cayenne peppers
    - *Cubanelle* peppers
    - Green chilies
    - *Habañero* peppers
    - *Jalapeño* peppers
    - Scotch bonnet chilies
    - Serrano peppers
    - Thai peppers
  - o Radicchio, raw

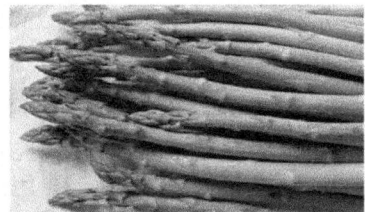

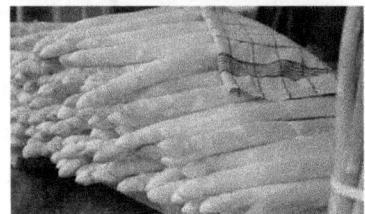

- o Radish, raw
- o Spinach, canned
- o Swiss chard, raw
- o Taro shoots, raw
- o Tomato
  - ▪ Tomato juice
- o Turnip greens or tops, raw
- o Winged beans, mature seeds, raw

8. To promote better health, the MTHFR diet recommends daily intake of dark leafy vegetables like arugula, kale, spinach and Swiss chard. Intake could be miniscule, or as little as ⅛ tsp. per meal, or as much as 3 cups per serving.

9. Increase consumption of food items high in organic zinc. These include:

- o Beans, lentils and peas (dried, canned, fresh, frozen)
  - ▪ Adzuki beans
  - ▪ Baked beans
  - ▪ Black eyed peas
  - ▪ Chickpeas
  - ▪ Kidney beans
  - ▪ Lentils
  - ▪ Lima beans
  - ▪ Peas (sparingly)
  - ▪ Soybeans (sparingly)
- o Cereals (sparingly)
  - ▪ Bran
  - ▪ Multi grain cereals
  - ▪ Whole grain cereals
- o Chocolate
  - ▪ Dark chocolate, unsweetened
  - ▪ Cocoa powder
- o Dairy (sparingly)
  - ▪ Cheese
    - • Brie
    - • Cheddar cheese (sparingly)
    - • Gouda
    - • Mozzarella

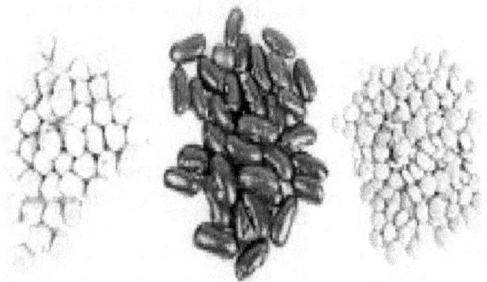

- - - Ricotta cheese
      - Swiss
    - Milk
      - Buttermilk (sparingly)
      - Skim
    - Yogurt, homemade
  - Eggs

  - Fruits
    - Avocadoes (sparingly)
    - Berries
      - Blackberries
      - loganberries
      - Raspberries
    - Dates
    - Pomegranates
  - Grains
    - Brown rice
    - Rice bran
    - Wheat germ
    - Wild rice, cooked
  - Meats
    - Beef (sparingly)
    - Chicken (sparingly)
    - Lamb (sparingly)
    - Turkey
  - Mushroom (sparingly)
    - Brown, raw
    - Morel, raw
    - Oyster, raw
    - Portabella, raw
    - Shiitake, raw
    - White mushroom (sparingly)
  - Nuts (sparingly)
    - Almonds
    - Cashew nuts
    - Hazelnuts

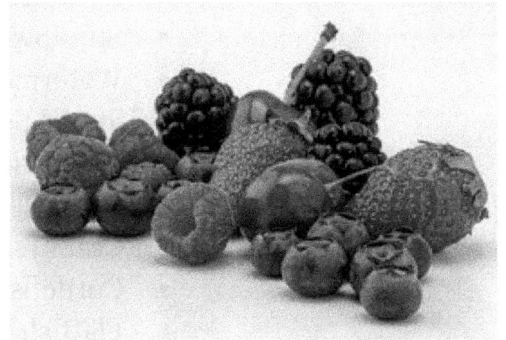

- Peanuts
- Peanut butter
- Pecan nuts
- Soy nuts
- Walnuts
  - Seeds
    - Flaxseeds
    - Pumpkin seeds (sparingly)
    - Sesame seeds (sparingly)
    - Squash seeds (sparingly)
    - Sunflower seeds
    - Watermelon seeds
  - Shellfish and Seafood
    - Anchovies (sparingly)
    - Clams (sparingly)
    - Crabs (sparingly)
    - Cuttlefish (sparingly)
    - Flatfish
    - Flounder
    - Lobsters (sparingly)
    - Mussels (sparingly)
    - Octopus (sparingly)
    - Oysters (sparingly)
    - Salmon (sparingly)
    - Scallops (sparingly)
    - Seaweed or kelp (sparingly)
    - Shrimps
    - Sole
  - Vegetables
    - Alfalfa sprouts
    - Asparagus (sparingly)
    - Brussels sprouts
    - Garlic
    - Green beans
    - Green peas
    - Hearts of palm
    - Napa cabbage
    - Pumpkin

- Spinach

10. If possible, lessen your daily consumption of food items high in folic acid.

Folic acid is not natural and appears in a lot of processed foods. Folate and Folinic Acid are natural and are essential for bone growth, but because many people who subscribe to the MTHFR diet cannot process *folic acid* properly, lessening your folic acid intake will make it easier for your digestion.

Food items high in natural folate are:
- Beans
  - Black beans
  - Green beans
  - Kidney beans
  - Lima beans
  - Navy beans
- Pinto beans Eggs and egg yolks
- Fruits
  - Avocado
  - Banana
  - Cantaloupe
  - Citrus fruits
  - Grapefruits
  - Limes
  - Oranges
  - Papayas
  - Raspberries
  - Strawberries
  - Guavas
  - Kiwi
  - Mangoes
  - Oranges
  - Peaches
  - Pomegranates
- Grains
  - Sweet potato
  - Wheat flour

- - Wholegrain bread
  - Lentils
  - Meat
    - Chicken giblets
    - Chicken kidney
    - Chicken Liver
  - Nuts
    - Almonds
    - Peanuts
  - Peas
    - Black-eyed peas
    - Chickpeas
    - Green peas
    - Split peas
  - Seeds
    - Flax seeds
    - Sunflower seeds
  - Vegetables, particularly leafy greens
    - Asparagus
    - Beets and beetroot
    - Broccoli
    - Brussels sprouts
    - Cauliflower
    - Carrots
    - Celery
    - Collard greens
    - Corn
    - Lettuce
      - Arugula
      - Butter head
      - Chicory
      - Cos
      - Endive
      - Romaine lettuce
      - Salad cress
      - Mustard greens
    - Okra
    - Squash

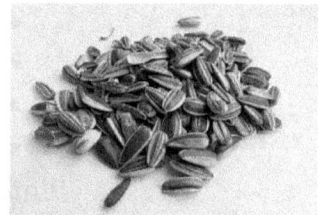

- Summer squash
  - Winter squash
  - Turnip greens

11. Limit or remove *purine*-rich food items from your diet.

All naturally-occurring food items contain *purine*, which is a chemical compound that carries the genetic structure of the source plant or animal. In small doses, *purine* acts as antioxidants which keep the blood's uric acid levels down.

However, because you are limiting your high purine protein intake with the MTHFR diet, it would be best to limit or remove *purine*-rich food. This is to prevent the destabilization of your uric acid, which can lead to: arthritis, gout, urinary tract infection, etc.

Limit your daily intake of:
- Grains, only ¼ cup or less per meal
  - Flavored, crushed, and/or instant oats
  - Rolled oats
- Fish and seafood, only 4 oz. or less per meal
  - Bluefish
  - Carp
  - Codfish
  - Crab
  - Halibut
  - Lobsters
  - Oysters
  - Perch
  - Salmon
  - Shellfish
  - Snapper
  - Trout
  - Tuna
- Legumes, only ¼ cup or less per meal
  - Kidney beans
  - Lentils
  - Lima bans

- o Navy beans
- o Peas
- Meat, only 4 oz. or less per meal
  - o Beef tongue and tripe
  - o Chicken liver
  - o Duck
  - o Goose
  - o Lamb and mutton
  - o Pork
  - o Rabbit
  - o Sheep
  - o Turkey
  - o Veal
  - o Venison
- Mushrooms, only ¼ cup or less per meal
- Vegetables, only ½ cup or less per meal
  - o Asparagus
  - o Cauliflower
  - o Spinach

Avoid consuming these:
- Canned or bottled anchovies
- Canned or bottled sardines
- Meat
  - o Beef kidney and liver
  - o Duck liver
  - o Goose liver
  - o Lamb liver
  - o Mutton liver
  - o Pork kidney and liver
  - o Rabbit liver
  - o Sheep liver
  - o Turkey liver
  - o Veal liver
- Store-bought bacon and ham
- Store-bought broths and stocks
- Store-bought chicken soups and stews
- Store-bought or instant gravies

- Sweetbreads, head cheese, and other cured meat using pork or beef "spare" parts (head, cheeks, internal organs, etc.)

12. Processed food should be removed completely from your daily meals, but you would still need a few ounces of fats and oils to carry flavor and for stir-frying.

Fats and oils are not necessarily bad for your health. Your body converts these into amino acids that make your hair look shiny, and your nails look pink and glossy. These amino acids also promote younger and elastic looking skin.

Use fats and oils sparingly. Some of the best sources are:

- Animal fat or lard, made from fresh produce, rendered fat
- Avocado oil
- Butter
    - Cultured butter or fermented butter
    - Ghee or clarified butter, homemade
    - Organic, raw or homemade
    - Whey butter
- Coconut oil
    - Centrifuged, cold pressed, expeller pressed
    - Homemade, fresh
    - Organic, dry milled, RBD (refined, bleached and deodorized)
    - Virgin, extra virgin, raw
- Flax oil or flaxseed oil (not to be used for cooking)
- Fish oil (not to be used for cooking)
    - Cod fish liver oil, not to be used for cooking but can be used as food supplement)
    - Tuna oil / roe, freshly rendered out, or consume with fresh fish
    - Salmon oil / roe, freshly rendered out, or consume with fresh fish
- Nut oils (only for low temperature cooking)
    - Macadamia nut oil
- Olive oil

- Extra virgin olive oil
- Pure olive oil
- Virgin olive oil
- Palm oil
  - Unrefined
- Peanut oil (only for low temperature cooking)

Avoid using:
- Animal fat or lard, commercially-made, store-bought
- Butter substitutes (overly-processed)
  - Ghee or clarified butter, commercial
- Coconut oil
  - Hydrogenated, partially hydrogenated, liquid coconut oil
  - Raw RBD (refined, bleached and deodorized,) Raw centrifuged
- Margarine
- Processed Olive oil
  - "Lite" or light olive oil
  - Refined olive oil
  - Olive *pomace* oil
- Vegetable lard (overly processed)
- Vegetable oils (though these contain good levels of Omega 3 and 6, these are processed with hexane solvent)
  - Canola oil
  - Corn oil
  - Cottonseed oil
  - Grape seed oil
  - Rapeseed oil
  - Rice bran oil
  - Safflower oil
  - Sesame oil
  - Soybean oil
  - Sunflower oil

You can also render out small amounts of oil in meat and nuts.

13. As an aid to digestion, add homemade, fermented and pickled food to your daily diet.

Fermented and pickled food items are not only great aids to digestion, but these make healthier alternatives to store-bought condiments, and commercial pickles. Some of the best ones to include in your daily meals are: sauerkraut, and pickled vegetables.

14. Eat small, whole fruits as snack, especially in between meals.

15. To speed up digestion, consume a cup of homemade meat or fish broth per meal.

16. When all else fails, practice moderation! Following any restrictive diet is hard. If you find yourself craving for food items that should not be in the MTHFR diet, just go ahead and take a bite – preferably a very small bite.

You do not have to go without your favorite food items and drinks all the time, but please practice moderation. And yes, find out the recommended portion per serving, and stick to that as well.

To make sure that you don't suffer too much from the consequences of consuming unhealthy food items and drinks, limit your diet "cheating" to once a week; one item only, and only within its own recommended meal or daily portion. So carefully read product labels, if any.

Chapter 2: 7 Day MTHFR Meal Plan

To make this diet diabetic-friendly, gluten-free, and easy for almost anyone's digestion, this meal plan follows the principle of consuming 5 to 6 small meals per day, with the last meal being entirely optional.

This kind of meal plan stabilizes insulin level quickly, and prevents you from feeling hungry during the day. This also promotes organic and gradual weight loss.

A few other tips to remember:

1. Never skip breakfast. After several hours without food, your blood will have an elevated insulin level. A small amount of food or drink in the morning will quickly stabilize your insulin level.

   If you regularly skip breakfast, you will automatically consume a lot once you start eating. Worse, you will also start craving for greasy, sweet, or salty food items during the rest of the day.

   In the same vein, never skip meals. Skipping meals will only destabilize your blood sugar level. This will only increase your chances of overindulging, and actually eating a lot in a short amount of time.

2. Schedule meals in regular 3-hour intervals. If you prefer breakfast early, or at 6 am, your mid-morning snack should be at 9 am, lunch at 12 noon, mid-afternoon snack at 3 pm, and dinner at 6 pm.

   Whatever schedule you prefer, make sure that your meals are evenly spaced out during the day.

3. Eat regularly on the same time each day. A regular eating pattern helps your body cope with your diet change. It also prevents your body from craving unwanted food items at odd hours of the day. If your body "knows" that it will be consuming something soon, it keeps hunger pangs and food cravings at bay.

4. Balance "light" snacks/meals and "heavy" snacks/meals evenly during the day. If you have "light" (uncooked) snacks in the morning, choose "heavy" (baked or cooked) snacks in the afternoon.

Likewise, if you are consuming heavier or protein-based meals in the morning, it would be best to limit your protein intake during lunch, and consume only vegetables during dinner. This makes it easier on your digestion.

This may also ease or prevent some or most of the symptoms of IBS or Irritable Bowel Syndrome.

5. Again, don't go full vegan. You need a few ounces of animal-based proteins daily. These do not have to be necessarily beef or pork based. You can eat consume a few ounces of white meat, fish, or eggs instead.

Plus, if you go full vegan, you need to take regular doses of B12 and other folate / folinic-based minerals to prevent your kidneys from failing. If you already have MTHFR mutation, this will only complicate matters and has to be dine correctly and under a knowledgeable physician's guidance.

Consume your daily dose of proteins. It's a far easier option.

6. Choose quality protein over higher quantity of protein every time. For example: eat the recommended 3 oz. of salmon, instead of consuming 2 cups of cashew nuts as snack.

Although cashew nuts are considered "healthier," eating 2 cups in one sitting is equivalent to consuming 24 grams of fat, while 3 oz. salmon only contains 11 grams of fat.

7. Except for red and white wine, skip alcoholic beverages (especially those that contain yeast) while you are on the MTHR diet. Use red and white wine for cooking.

This is an example of a 7-day MTHFR meal plan.
* Note: if ingredients or recommended meals are in bold letters, then the recipes are contained within the book.

Sunday
Breakfast:

1	cup	**Roasted Beef Broth**
1	stack	**Banana Flapjacks**
-	-	**Homemade Yogurt**
-	-	drinking water, as much as you want

Mid-Morning Snack:

1	cup	**Vegetable Broth**
½	cup	gluten-free crackers, store-bought
1	piece, large	apple
-	-	drinking water, as much as you want

Lunch:

1	cup	**Fish Broth**
-	-	**Fresh Salad with Quail Eggs and Apple Cider Vinaigrette**
-	-	**Homemade Quick Ferment *Kimchi***
-	-	drinking water, as much as you want

Mid-Day Snack:

1	cup	**Chicken Broth**
¼	cup	roasted watermelon or pumpkin seeds
-	-	drinking water, as much as you want

Early Dinner:

1	cup	**Light Veal Broth**
-	-	**Colorful Asian-Inspired Chicken Salad**
-	-	**Colorful Pickled Vegetables**
-	-	drinking water, as much as you want

Final Snack: (optional)

1	cup	**Fresh Fruit Salad**

Monday

Breakfast:

1	cup	**Light Chicken Broth**
-	-	**Sweet Boiled Plantains**
-	-	**Homemade Kefir**
-	-	drinking water, as much as you want

Mid-Morning Snack:

1	cup	**Dark Pork Broth**
1	piece, large	apricot
-	-	drinking water, as much as you want

Lunch:

1	cup	**Shrimp Broth**
-	-	**Ground Chicken and Mushrooms in Lettuce Wraps**
-	-	**Homemade Pickled Green Papaya**
-	-	drinking water, as much as you want

Mid-Day Snack:

1	cup	**Roasted Vegetable Broth**
½	cup	raisins
-	-	drinking water, as much as you want

Early Dinner:

1	cup	**Fish Broth**
-	-	**Beef Stroganoff with Zucchini Pasta**
-	-	**Homemade Picked Cucumber**
-	-	drinking water, as much as you want

Final Snack: (optional)

1	piece, large	banana

Tuesday

Breakfast:

1	cup	**Dark Chicken Broth**
-	-	**Steel-Cut Oats with Toasted Walnuts and Assorted Berries**
-	-	**Homemade Yogurt**
-	-	drinking water, as much as you want

Mid-Morning Snack:

1	cup	**Roasted Vegetable Broth**
1	piece, large	custard apple or *cherimoya*
-	-	drinking water, as much as you want

Lunch:

1	cup	**Light Lamb Broth**
-	-	**Grilled Cheesy Mushroom Sandwich**
-	-	**Homemade Quick Ferment *Kimchi***
-	-	drinking water, as much as you want

Mid-Day Snack:

1	cup	**Shrimp Broth**
1	cup	fresh strawberries with
½	cup	whipped cream
-	-	drinking water, as much as you want

Early Dinner:

1	cup	**Fish Broth**
-	-	**Baked Salmon Fillets with Kale Chips**
-	-	**Colorful Pickled Vegetables**
-	-	drinking water, as much as you want

Final Snack: (optional)

-	-	**Creamy Banana Slurry**

Wednesday

Breakfast:

1	cup	**Roasted Beef Broth**
-	-	**Warm Steel-Cut Oats with Almond Milk and Avocado**
-	-	**Homemade Kefir**
-	-	drinking water, as much as you want

Mid-Morning Snack:

1	cup	**Vegetable Broth**
½	cup	fresh roasted walnuts
-	-	drinking water, as much as you want

Lunch:

1	cup	**Fish Broth**
-	-	**No Cook Spicy Curry Tuna Salad in Lettuce Wraps**
-	-	**Homemade Pickled Cucumber**
-	-	drinking water, as much as you want

Mid-Day Snack:

1	cup	**Chicken Broth**
1	piece, large	apple
-	-	drinking water, as much as you want

Early Dinner:

1	cup	**Light Veal Broth**
-	-	**Quick Fry Chicken with Cauliflower and Water Chestnuts on Wild Rice**
-	-	**Homemade Pickled Green Papaya**
-	-	drinking water, as much as you want

Final Snack: (optional)

| 1 | slice, small | **Coconut Cream Pie** |

Thursday

Breakfast:

1	cup	**Dark Chicken Broth**
-	-	**Sweet Banana-Cashew Flapjacks**
-	-	**Homemade Yogurt**
-	-	drinking water, as much as you want

Mid-Morning Snack:

1	cup	**Roasted Vegetable Broth**
¼	cup	toasted pistachio nuts, lightly salted
-	-	drinking water, as much as you want

Lunch:

1	cup	**Light Lamb Broth**
-	-	**Roasted Carrots Salad with Cashew, Cottage Cheese and Spinach**
-	-	**Homemade Traditional _Kimchi_**
-	-	drinking water, as much as you want

Mid-Day Snack:

1	cup	**Shrimp Broth**
1	piece, large	pear
-	-	drinking water, as much as you want

Early Dinner:

1	cup	**Fish Broth**
-	-	**Oatmeal Crusted Chicken Wings and Vegetables**
-	-	**Homemade Traditional Sauerkraut**
-	-	drinking water, as much as you want

Final Snack: (optional)

-	-	**Creamy Banana Slurry**

Friday

Breakfast:

1	cup	**Roasted Beef Broth**
1	piece	**Almond Meal Muffin**
-	-	**Homemade Kefir**
-	-	drinking water, as much as you want

Mid-Morning Snack:

1	cup	**Vegetable Broth**
½	cup	fresh roasted pecan nuts
-	-	drinking water, as much as you want

Lunch:

1	cup	**Fish Broth**
-	-	**Three Cheese Grilled Sandwich**
-	-	**Homemade Quick Pickled Cucumber**
-	-	drinking water, as much as you want

Mid-Day Snack:

1	cup	**Chicken Broth**
¼	cup	fresh blueberries
-	-	drinking water, as much as you want

Early Dinner:

1	cup	**Light Veal Broth**
-	-	**Steamed Meat Log**
-	-	**Colorful Pickled Vegetables**
-	-	drinking water, as much as you want

Final Snack: (optional)

-	-	**Watermelon and Lime Ice Lollies**

Saturday
Breakfast:

1	cup	**Light Chicken Broth**
-	-	**Assorted Berry Juice**
-	-	**Homemade Yogurt** with
1	piece, large	banana, preferably overripe, roughly chopped, and
¼	cup	assorted fresh berries of choice
-	-	drinking water, as much as you want

Mid-Morning Snack:

1	cup	**Dark Pork Broth**
1	piece, large	apricot
-	-	drinking water, as much as you want

Lunch:

1	cup	**Shrimp Broth**
-	-	**Pan-Fried Aubergine and Tomato with Mozzarella and Homemade Feta**
-	-	**Colorful Pickled Vegetables**
-	-	drinking water, as much as you want

Mid-Day Snack:

1	cup	**Roasted Vegetable Broth**
½	cup	raisins
-	-	drinking water, as much as you want

Early Dinner:

1	cup	**Fish Broth**
-	-	**Pan-Fried Tuna Steaks with Spicy Cauliflower Pops**
-	-	**Homemade Traditional Sauerkraut**

-       -   drinking water, as much as you want

Final Snack: (optional)

-       -   **Exotic Fresh Fruit Salad**

Chapter 3: Breakfast Recipes

* Note: if ingredients are in bold letters, then the recipes are contained within the book.

Recipe #1: Banana Flapjacks
Yields 8 small flapjacks, recommended serving size: stack of 2 small flapjacks per meal

Ingredients:

2	pieces, large	eggs, lightly beaten
1	piece, large	banana, preferably overripe, roughly mashed, leave a few larger chunks for texture
-	-	cooking oil, for greasing

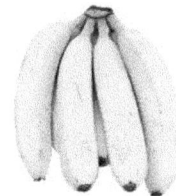

You will also need:

-	-	non-stick frying pan or griddle

Directions:

1. Lightly grease a non-stick frying pan set over medium heat.
2. Whisk eggs and mashed banana together. Batter should look chunky and watery. Divide into 8 equal portions.
3. Pour individual portions on hot frying pan. Flapjacks are done when edges are set and golden, but center is still wobbly, about 1 to 2 minutes.
4. Gently flip and cook other side for another minute.
5. Stack cooked pancakes on a serving plate. Keep warm until ready to serve.

Recipe #2: Sweet Banana-Cashew Flapjacks
Yields 8 small flapjacks, recommended serving size: stack of 2 small flapjacks per meal

Ingredients:

2	pieces, large	eggs, lightly beaten
2	pieces, large	banana, preferably overripe, roughly mashed, leave a few larger chunks for texture
1	pinch, generous	raw cashew, shelled, halved lengthwise, roughly chopped
-	dash	nutmeg powder
-	drop	vanilla extract

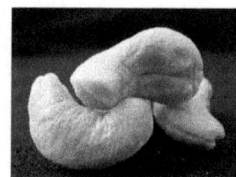

You will also need:

| - | - | non-stick frying pan or griddle |

Directions:

1. Place raw cashew in a non-stick frying pan set over high heat. Toast nuts while stirring often. Nuts are done when cashew gives off nutty smell, and look golden and waxy. Set aside. Divide into 8 equal portions.
2. Whisk remaining ingredients together. Divide into 8 equal portions.
3. Pour individual portions on the same frying pan. Flapjacks are done when edges are set and golden, but center is still wobbly, about 1 minute.
4. Sprinkle equal portions of toasted cashew nuts in the wobbly center.
5. Gently flip and cook other side for another minute.
6. Stack cooked pancakes on a serving plate. Keep warm until ready to serve.

Recipe #3: Steel-Cut Oats with Toasted Walnuts and Assorted Berries
Yields 2 cups, recommended serving size: ½ cups cooked plus 1 heaping tablespoon of walnut-berry sauce per meal

Ingredients:

For the oat base

1	cup	water, add more only if needed
1	cup	milk of choice, divided (substitute almond milk, if desired)
1	cup	steel-cut oats
-	dash	nutmeg powder
-	drop	vanilla extract

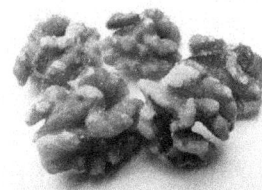

For the walnut-berry sauce

½	cup	raw walnut, shelled, roughly chopped
½	cup	water
¼	cup	fresh or frozen raspberries
¼	cup	fresh or frozen blueberries
¼	cup	fresh or frozen cranberries
¼	cup	fresh or frozen strawberries
1	Tbsp., heaping	raisins
1	tsp.	*stevia*
1	tsp.	lemon juice, preferably fresh-squeezed

You will also need:

| 2 | pieces | deep, heavy-bottomed sauce pans |
| 1 | piece | non-stick skillet |

Directions:

1. <u>To prepare oats</u>: except for vanilla extract, pour all ingredients in a sauce pan set over medium heat. Let this come to a soft boil.
2. Immediately turn down heat to lowest setting. Partially put lid on. Let oats cook for 15 to 20 minutes, stirring often. Oats should be runny. Add more water, if needed.
3. Remove sauce pan from heat. Add in vanilla extract. Stir. Let oats cool slightly, uncovered.

4. <u>To prepare walnut-berry sauce</u>: toast walnuts in skillet set over medium heat. Shake skillet often. Walnuts are done when these become aromatic and slightly deeper in color. Set aside.

5. Except for *stevia* and lemon juice, add remaining ingredients of walnut-berry sauce in another sauce pan set over medium heat.
6. Let this come to a full boil while stirring often. Mash berries lightly to release more flavor.
7. Cook until sauce is reduced and thickened, about 3 to 5 minutes.
8. Stir in *stevia* and lemon juice.

9. <u>To assemble</u>: ladle ½ cup of cooked oats into a small bowl.
10. Drizzle 1 tablespoon of the berry sauce on top.
11. Sprinkle a pinch of toasted walnuts on top. Serve immediately.

Recipe #4: Warm Steel-Cut Oats with Almond Milk and Avocado (Beverage)
Yields 2 cups, recommended serving size: 1 cup per meal

Ingredients:

1	cup	water
½	cup	almond milk, or any dairy-based drink of choice, add more if desired
¼	cup	steel-cut oats
½	piece	ripe avocado, pitted, skin peeled
1	tsp.	*stevia*

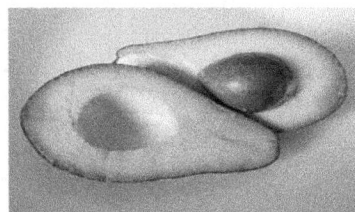

You will also need:

1	piece	sauce pan
-	-	blender or food processor

Directions:

1. Place water and steel-cut oats in saucepan set over medium heat.
2. Let water come to a soft boil. Turn down heat to lowest setting. Let oats cook for 20 minutes, stirring often.
3. Immediately remove saucepan from heat. Allow oats to cool slightly before pouring into blender.
4. Add in remaining ingredients into blender.
5. Process beverage until smooth. Check consistency of beverage. If it is too thick, add more milk. Process once more until smooth.
6. Pour equal portions into cups. Serve while warm.

Recipe #5: Assorted Berry Juice (Beverage)
Yields 2 cups, recommended serving size: 1 cup per meal

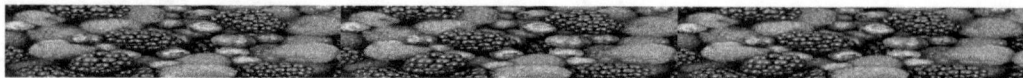

Ingredients:

1	cup	ice shavings or crushed ice
3	pieces, large	frozen strawberries, halved
1	piece, large	frozen overripe banana, roughly chopped
¼	cup	frozen blueberries
¼	cup	frozen blackberries
¼	cup	frozen raspberries

You will also need:

-	-	blender or food processor
-	-	fine-meshed sieve or strainer

Directions:

1. Add all ingredients into blender.
2. Process until smooth.
3. Pour equal portions into glasses through a sieve. Serve immediately.

Recipe #6: Assorted Fresh Fruit Juice (Beverage)
Yields 2 cups, recommended serving size: 1 cup per meal

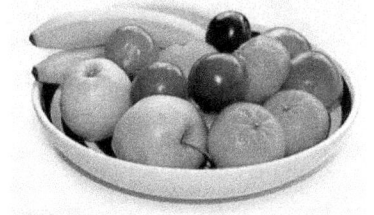

Ingredients:

1	cup	ice shavings or crushed ice
¼	cup	frozen grapes, pitted, halved
1	can, 8 oz.	crushed pineapple or pineapple tidbits, drained
¼	cup	grape or prune juice
1	piece, large	frozen overripe banana, roughly chopped
1	piece, small	apple, cored, roughly chopped

You will also need:

-	-	blender or food processor

Directions:

1. Add all ingredients into blender.
2. Process until smooth.
3. Pour equal portions into glasses. Serve immediately.

Recipe #7: Apple and Carrots Milkshake (Beverage)
Yields 2 cups, recommended serving size: 1 cup per meal

Ingredients:

1	cup	ice shavings or crushed ice
½	cup	cold milk, or any dairy substitute of choice
1	piece, large	apple, cored, roughly chopped
1	piece, medium	carrot, top removed, roughly chopped
1	tsp.	*stevia* (optional)

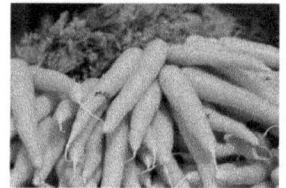

You will also need:

-	-	blender or food processor

Directions:

1. Add all ingredients into blender.
2. Process until smooth.
3. Pour equal portions into tall glasses. Serve immediately.

Recipe #8: Sweet Boiled Plantains
Yields 8 plantains, recommended serving size: 2 pieces per meal

Ingredients:

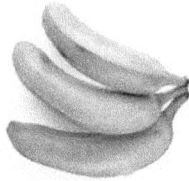

| 8 | pieces, medium | very overripe plantains, trim but do not remove stems, scrub skins (Use *Benedetta* banana, *Cardaba* Banana, *Saba,* or any plantain variety with thick skins, as these usually have the sweetest flavors. But any overripe plantain will do.) |
| - | - | water, enough to cover plantains in cooking pot |

You will also need:

| - | - | cooking pot, large enough to hold all plantains and water |
| - | - | colander or strainer |

Directions:

1. Place all plantains into cooking pot.
2. Cover with just enough water to fully submerge plantains.
3. Set cooking pot over high heat. Let water come to a full boil.
4. Turn down heat to lowest setting. Put lid partially on. Boil plantains for 15 minutes.
5. After 15 minutes, carefully strain out boiled plantains. Plantains and cooking liquid may turn purplish, but that is normal. Allow to cool slightly before serving.
6. To serve: remove skins of 2 plantains, and place flesh on a plate. Serve.

Or

7. If you are packing this for lunch or as a snack, keep skins on until you are ready to eat. Consume as you would a (very overripe and wobbly) banana.

Note: grocers and fruit vendors usually do not sell overripe plantains. Buy your green or semi-ripe plantains, and let these ripen at home. Do not place in fridge.

Recipe #9: *Arroz a la Cubana* (Heavier Breakfast Option)
Yields 6 cups, recommended serving size: ½ cup rice, ¼ cup filling, 1 piece egg, and ½ piece plantain per meal

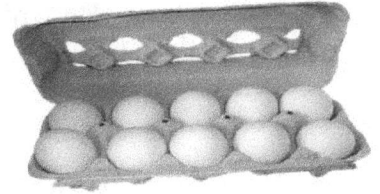

Ingredients:

6	pieces, small	eggs (smallest chicken eggs you can find)
3	pieces, small	plantain, semi-ripe or ripe, skins removed, halved lengthwise
1½	cups	brown or wild rice, cooked according to package instructions, fluff up grains using a fork, divide into 6 equal portions
-	-	sea or kosher salt, to taste
-	-	oil, for greasing frying pan

For the filling

½	pound	ground beef, 90% lean
½	pound	ground pork, 90% lean
½	cup	frozen peas, thawed, drained well
¼	cup	raisins
1	clove, large	garlic, minced
1	piece, large	white onion, minced
1½	Tbsp.	tomato puree
1½	Tbsp.	tomato sauce
1½	Tbsp.	Worcestershire sauce
½	Tbsp.	sea or kosher salt

-	dash	black pepper, to taste
1	piece	bird's eye chili, minced (optional)
-	-	oil, for greasing frying pan

You will also need:

-	-	large non-stick skillet or frying pan
-	-	smaller non-stick skillet or frying pan
2	pieces	plates

Directions:

1. <u>To make filling</u>: spray small amount of oil into skillet set over medium heat. Add in onion and garlic. Stir-fry until former is limp and transparent.
2. Add in meat. Stir-fry while breaking up clumps, about 2 minutes.
3. Add in remaining ingredients. Stir-fry for another minute. Turn down heat, and let filling cook for 10 to 15 minutes, or until juices are greatly reduced. Stir often.
4. Taste. Add more seasoning only if needed.
5. Turn off heat. Divide into 6 equal portions.

6. <u>To prepare eggs</u>: spray small amount of oil into smaller skillet set over medium heat. Cook eggs sunny-side up, one piece at a time. Lightly season with salt. Transfer to holding plate.

7. <u>To prepare plantains</u>: spray a little more oil into same skillet. Fry plantain halves until golden on both sides.

8. <u>To assemble</u>: place 1 portion of rice on a plate, along with 1 portion of filling, 1 egg and a fried plantain half. Serve while warm.

Recipe #10: Almond Meal Muffins
Yields 10 muffins, recommended serving size: 1 muffin per meal

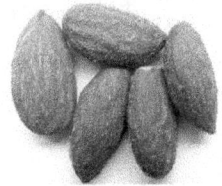

Ingredients:

1	cup	almond meal, preferably ground fresh from raw almonds using food processor
¾	cup	steel-cut oats, ground fine using food processor
¼	cup	oil, any mild tasting cooking oil will do
2	pieces, small	eggs at room temperature, separate whites and yolks
2	pieces, medium	bananas, preferably overripe, mashed well
3	Tbsp.	*stevia,* or any baking sweetener of choice
3	Tbsp.	almond milk, or any dairy substitute of choice
1	tsp.	vanilla extract

Garnishes (optional)

1	piece, large	banana, thinly sliced into 20 disks
-	dollop, each	store-bought whipped cream, well-chilled

You will also need:

-	-	blender or food processor
2	pieces, large	large bowl
-	-	muffin tins
-	-	paper liners

		whisk
-	-	rubber spatula
-	-	cooling rack
-	-	

Directions:

1. Preheat oven to 350°F or 175°C. Place paper liners in muffin tins.
2. Place egg whites in large mixing bowl. Using food processor with whisk attachment, process until stiff peaks form. Set aside.
3. In another large bowl, whisk in remaining ingredients. Mix well.
4. Using a rubber spatula, **gently** fold in egg whites.
5. Spoon batter into paper liners, filling each ¾ full.
6. Bake muffins for 25 to 30 minutes, or until toothpick inserted in center comes out clean.
7. Remove muffin tin from oven. Set on cooling rack and let cool for 5 minutes.
8. After 5 minutes, carefully remove muffins from tin. Set on cooling rack. Let these cool completely to room temperature before garnishing.

9. <u>To assemble</u>: place a dollop of whipped cream, and two slices of banana on top of each muffin. Serve.

Recipe #11: Fresh Salad with Quail Eggs and Apple Cider Vinaigrette
Yields 4 cups, recommended serving size: 2 generous cups fresh greens, 3 quail eggs, and 1½ Tbsp. dressing per meal

Ingredients:

For the fresh salad

1	head, large	iceberg lettuce, cored, roughly torn, rinsed, spun-dry
1	head, large	Romaine lettuce, cored, roughly torn, rinsed, spun-dry
1	head, large	watercress, cored, roughly torn, rinsed, spun-dry
1	bag, 5 oz. each	baby spinach, roughly chopped, rinsed, spun-dry
6	pieces	quail eggs, boiled, shelled
1	piece, small	carrot, julienned
1	piece, small	radish, finely shaved (use mandolin or vegetable peeler)

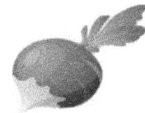

For the apple-cider vinaigrette

3	Tbsp.	apple cider vinegar, preferably sugar-free
1	tsp.	yellow mustard (substitute English mustard for spicier mix)
-	dash	sea or kosher salt
-	dash	white pepper powder (optional)
-	dash	red pepper flakes (optional)

You will also need:

1	piece	air-tight container, just large enough for the dressing
-	-	large salad bowl for mixing

Directions:

1. <u>To make the dressing</u>: combine all ingredients of dressing in a small air-tight container. Shake well. Chill until ready to use.

2. <u>To make salad</u>: Except for quail eggs, toss salad ingredients well in large salad bowl.

3. If you are serving immediately, pour dressing into the greens. Toss well to combine. Divide into 2 equal portions.
4. Dot surface with equal amounts of quail eggs. Serve.

Or

5. If you are packing this for lunch, place salad greens and quail eggs in one container, and dressing into another.
6. Combine only when you are ready to eat. Toss. Serve.

Recipe #12: Spinach Salad with Strawberry Vinaigrette
Yields 4 servings, recommended serving size: 2 cups fresh spinach, and ¼ cup of dressing per meal

Ingredients:

For the fresh salad

2	bags, 5 oz. each	baby spinach, roughly chopped, rinsed, spun-dry
¼	cup (do not pack)	homemade cottage cheese (no rennet,) crumbled (See recipe on page yyy)
¼	cup	raw cashew nuts, roughly chopped freshly toasted

For the strawberry vinaigrette

¾	cup	fresh strawberries, hulled, quartered
4	leaves, large	fresh basil, minced
2	Tbsp.	white wine vinegar
1	Tbsp.	extra virgin olive oil
-	dash	sea or kosher salt
-	dash	white pepper

You will also need:

-	-	large salad bowl for mixing
-	-	blender or food processor

Directions:

1. <u>To make the dressing</u>: combine all ingredients of dressing in a blender. Process until smooth. Chill before using.
2. <u>To make salad</u>: toss salad ingredients well in large salad bowl.

3. If you are serving immediately, pour dressing into greens. Toss well to combine. Divide into 4 equal portions. Serve.

Or

4. If you are packing this for lunch, place equal portions of salad greens in separate containers, and dressings into separate bottle.
5. Combine only when you are ready to eat. Toss. Serve.

Recipe #13: Ground Chicken and Mushrooms in Lettuce Wraps
Yields 8 wraps, recommended serving size: 2 wraps with ¼ pound filling per meal

Ingredients:

8	leaves, large	fresh Boston or iceberg lettuce, rinsed spun-dry, chilled before using

For filling

¾	pound	ground chicken, preferably 90% lean (substitute leftover boiled/roasted chicken, shredded or minced)
3	Tbsp.	fish sauce
1	Tbsp.	olive oil
1	Tbsp.	white vinegar
1	Tbsp.	**Homemade Catsup**
1	tsp.	sesame oil, add more only if needed
1	tsp.	ginger, freshly-grated
1	can, 8 oz.	water chestnuts, rinsed well, drain, minced
1	clove, large	garlic, minced
2	pieces, large	fresh Portabella mushrooms, roots trimmed, thinly sliced
1	piece, small	carrot, julienned
1	piece, small	shallot, minced

You will also need:

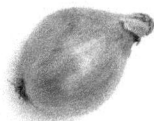

-                   -   non-stick skillet or frying pan
-                   -   small plate

Directions:

1. Pour 1 tablespoon oil into skillet set over medium heat. Wait for oil to become slightly smoky before searing mushrooms.
2. Brown mushrooms on both sides, about 1 minute each. Do not crowd skillet, or mushrooms will render out too much moisture. Brown mushrooms in batches, if necessary. Transfer mushrooms to a plate. Set aside.

3. In same skillet, add in ground chicken and onions. (Add a tablespoon of oil only if pan looks too dry.)
4. Stir-fry until raw chicken is no longer pink. Break apart large clumps, if any. (If you are using leftover meat, cook until onions are limp and transparent.)
5. Except for sesame oil, add in remaining ingredients into skillet. Stir-fry until sauce thickens, about 5 to 7 minutes (or less.)
6. Remove skillet from heat. Let filling cool slightly before serving.

7. <u>To serve</u>: spoon equal portions of filling into 8 lettuce leaves. Serve immediately.

Recipe #14: No Cook Spicy Curry Tuna Salad in Lettuce Wraps
Yields 6 wraps, recommended serving size: 3 wraps with 1 heaping teaspoon of filling in each wrap, per meal

Ingredients:

6	leaves, large	fresh Green Leaf, Romaine or Batavia lettuce, rinsed spun-dry, chilled before using (substitute any lettuce variety with upright spine)

For the onion pickle

1	piece, small	shallot, thinly sliced
1	pinch	sea or kosher salt

For filling

1	can, 5 oz.	tuna chunks in water or brine, drained lightly, reserve…
1	Tbsp.	tuna brine
1	Tbsp.	**Homemade Greek yogurt**
1	Tbsp.	English or Russian mustard
-	dash	sea or kosher salt
-	dash	white pepper
-	dash	Spanish or sweet paprika
-	dash	curry powder
1	piece, small	green chili, deseeded, minced (optional)

You will also need:

-       -   large mixing bowl
-       -   small mixing bowl
-       -   fine-meshed strainer

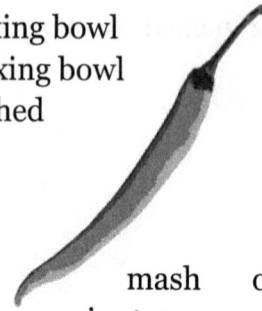

Directions:

1. <u>To make onion pickle</u>: using your fingers, mash onion slices and salt in a small bowl. Set aside for 15 minutes, uncovered.
2. After 15 minutes, rinse onions under running water. Drain well using a strainer. Set aside until ready to use.

3. <u>To make tuna filling</u>: combine all ingredients in a large bowl. Taste.
4. Adjust seasoning, if needed. Chill well before using.

5. <u>To assemble</u>: spread generous teaspoon of filling along inner spine of each lettuce leaf. Serve immediately.

As variation: instead of 3 filled lettuce leaves, use:

½	thin slice, toasted	wholegrain or multi-grain bread, with
1	tsp.	tuna filling

Recipe #15: Crunchy Tuna Salad in Lettuce Wraps
Yields 6 wraps, recommended serving size: 3 wraps with 1 heaping teaspoon of filling in each wrap, per meal

Ingredients:

6	leaves, large	fresh iceberg lettuce, rinse, spun-dry

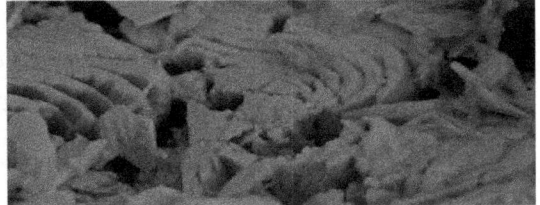

For filling

1	can, 5 oz.	tuna chunks in water or brine, drained
1	piece, medium	shallot, minced
1	piece, small	carrot, finely grated, juice squeezed out
1	Tbsp.	**Homemade Greek Yogurt**
1	Tbsp.	English or Russian mustard
1	Tbsp., heaping	raw cashew, freshly roasted on a dry pan
1	Tbsp., heaping	raisins
-	-	sea or kosher salt, to taste
-	-	white pepper, to taste
-	dash	Spanish or sweet paprika

You will also need:

large mixing bowl

Directions:

1. <u>To make filling</u>: combine all ingredients in a large bowl. Taste.
2. Adjust seasoning, if needed. Chill well before using. Divide filling into 6 equal portions.

3. <u>To assemble</u>: spoon 1 portion of filling into each lettuce leaf. Roll, fold, or pinch leaf edges together. Serve immediately.

Recipe #16: Pan-Fried Aubergine and Tomato with Mozzarella and Homemade Feta

Yields 2 stacks, recommended serving size: 1 stack per meal

Ingredients:

1	piece, medium	firm tomato, top and bottom removed, sliced thickly into 2 thick disks
2	pieces, large	fresh basil leaves, minced, divided
1	piece, large	aubergine, tops and bottoms removed, sliced thickly into 4 disks, divided
2	balls, small	buffalo mozzarella, roughly torn, divided
2	tsp.	**Homemade Feta Cheese**
-	-	salt, to taste
-	-	black pepper, to taste
-	-	oil, for frying

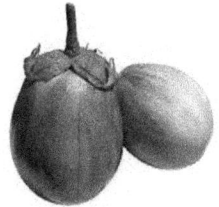

You will also need:

-	-	non-stick skillet or frying pan

Directions:

1. Spray small amount of oil into skillet set over medium heat.
2. Fry aubergine slices in batches until golden brown on both sides, about 5 minutes. Transfer to holding plate.
3. Fry tomato slices in batches until seared on both sides, about 5 minutes.

4. <u>To assemble</u>: stack your salad starting with an aubergine base, torn buffalo mozzarella, minced basil leaves, tomato slice, and then ½ teaspoon of feta cheese.
5. Top of with another slice of aubergine and another ½ tsp of feta cheese.
6. Stack the other salad similarly. Serve.

Recipe #17: Roasted Carrots Salad with Cashew, Cottage Cheese and Spinach
Yields 6 servings, recommended serving size: 2 cups per meal

Ingredients:

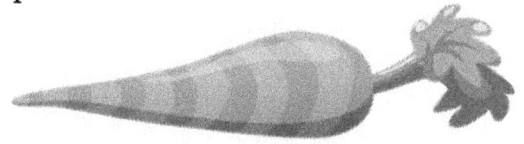

For roasted carrots

2	pieces, large	carrots, cubed into bite-sized pieces
½	Tbsp.	olive oil
½	cup	raw cashew nuts, halved lengthwise
2	tsp.	cumin powder
-	-	salt, to taste
-	-	black pepper, to taste

For lemon vinaigrette

1	piece, large	lemon, juiced
1	Tbsp.	*stevia*
1	tsp.	extra virgin olive oil
-	-	salt, to taste
-	-	black pepper, to taste

For the salad greens

| 2 | bags, 5 oz. each | baby spinach, roughly chopped, rinsed, spun-dry |
| 2 | bags, 5 oz. each | arugula, roughly chopped, rinsed, spun-dry (substitute assorted salad greens, if desired) |

For the garnish

| ½ | cup, loosely packed | **Homemade Cottage Cheese**, divided into 6 equal portions, crumbled |

You will also need:

-	-	baking sheet
-	-	parchment paper
2	pieces	bowls, for mixing
1	piece	large salad bowl, for tossing

Directions:

1. <u>For roasting carrots</u>: preheat oven to 400°F or 200°C for at least 5 minutes. Line a baking sheet with parchment paper.
2. Combine all ingredients in a bowl. Mix until everything is coated in oil.
3. Place baking sheet in oven. Roast carrots for 25 to 30 minutes, or until fork-tender. Cashew nuts should look golden brown. Remove baking sheet from oven. Let cool completely to room temperature before using.

4. <u>For lemon vinaigrette</u>: in separate bowl, combine all ingredients. Adjust seasoning according to personal taste.
5. Drizzle 1 teaspoon over cooked carrots. Toss well to combine. Set aside.

6. Combine salad greens and roasted vegetables in large salad bowl. Toss well to combine.
7. If serving immediately, drizzle in remaining vinaigrette. Divide into 6 equal portions. Plate.
8. Garnish with 1 portion of cottage cheese. Serve.

Or

9. If serving later, place fresh greens, roasted vegetables, and cottage cheese in 1 container, and vinaigrette in another.
10. Drizzle in vinaigrette when you are ready to eat. Toss well. Serve.

Recipe #18: Grilled Cheesy Mushroom Sandwich
Yields 2 servings, recommended serving size: ½ sandwich per meal

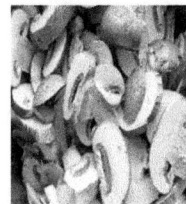

Ingredients:

| 2 | slices, thick | wholegrain or whole wheat bread (choose organic,) lightly toasted |
| ½ | tsp. | **Homemade Garlic and Parsley Butter**, leave out early so spreading is easier |

Filling

1	can, 15 oz.	canned button or portabella mushrooms, stems and pieces, rinsed, drained well, divided
2	Tbsp.	**Homemade Cottage Cheese**, crumbled
2	balls, small	buffalo mozzarella, roughly shredded, divided
4	stalks	fresh parsley, minced

You will also need:

-	-	stove-top non-stick skillet or electric grill
-	-	small mixing bowl
-	-	heat-proof chopping board

Directions:
1. Place skillet over medium heat. If using an electric grill, preheat machine before using.
2. Combine filling ingredients in a small bowl. Set aside.
3. Pat butter on all sides of bread. Spread thinly.

4. Spread filling on 1 bread slice. Top off with other slice. Press down slightly.
5. Place sandwich on grill. Sear both sides until golden, and mozzarella is runny.
6. Remove sandwich from grill, and place on cutting board. Halve diagonally.
7. Plate. Serve while warm.

Recipe #19: Three Cheese Grilled Sandwich

Yields 2 servings, recommended serving size: ½ sandwich per meal

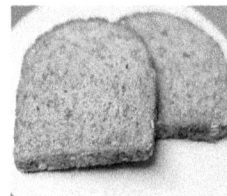

Ingredients:

| 2 | slices, thick | wholegrain or whole wheat bread (choose organic,) lightly toasted |
| ½ | tsp. | **Homemade Pizza-Flavored Butter**, leave out early so spreading is easier |

Filling

1	Tbsp., heaping	shallot, finely sliced
1	Tbsp., level	bell or sweet pepper, minced
1	Tbsp.	**Homemade Feta Cheese**, divided into 6 equal portions
1	Tbsp.	Colby Jack cheese, store-bought, grated
2	balls, small	buffalo mozzarella, roughly shredded, divided

You will also need:

-	-	stove-top non-stick skillet or electric grill
-	-	small mixing bowl
-	-	heat-proof chopping board

Directions:

1. Place skillet over medium heat. If using an electric grill, preheat machine before using.
2. Combine filling ingredients in a small bowl. Set aside.
3. Pat butter on all sides of bread. Spread thinly.
4. Spread filling on 1 bread slice. Top off with other slice. Press down slightly.
5. Place sandwich on grill. Sear both sides until golden, and mozzarella is runny.
6. Remove sandwich from grill, and place on cutting board. Halve diagonally.
7. Plate. Serve while warm.

Recipe #20: Spicy Avocado and Cheese Grilled Sandwich
Yields 2 servings, recommended serving size: ½ sandwich per meal

Ingredients:

2	slices, thick	wholegrain or whole wheat bread (choose organic,) lightly toasted
½	tsp.	**Homemade Cilantro and Lime Butter**, leave out early so spreading is easier

Filling

1	Tbsp.	Pepper Jack cheese, store-bought, grated
1	Tbsp.	cheddar cheese, store-bought, grated
2	balls, small	buffalo mozzarella, roughly shredded, divided
4	stalks, small	cilantro, minced

You will also need:

-	-	stove-top non-stick skillet or electric grill
-	-	small mixing bowl
-	-	heat-proof chopping board

Directions:

1. Place skillet over medium heat. If using an electric grill, preheat machine before using.
2. Combine filling ingredients in a small bowl. Set aside.
3. Pat butter on all sides of bread. Spread thinly.
4. Spread filling on 1 bread slice. Top off with other slice. Press down slightly.
5. Place sandwich on grill. Sear both sides until golden, and mozzarella is runny.

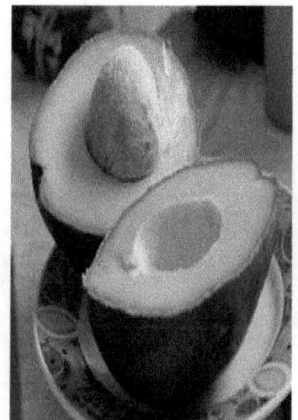

6. Remove sandwich from grill, and place on cutting board. Halve diagonally.
7. Plate. Serve while warm.

Chapter 5: Indulgent Dinner Recipes

Recipe #21: Colorful Asian-Inspired Chicken Salad
Yields 2 servings, recommended serving size: 1½ cup per meal

Ingredients:

For salad

3	cups	cooked chicken, (roasted, broiled, or boiled leftovers are fine,) shredded
¼	cup	raw cashew nuts, freshly roasted on dry pan
1	handful	cilantro leaves, roughly torn
1	can, 8 oz.	crushed pineapple, or pineapple tidbit drained
1	piece, large	carrot, julienned
1	piece, small	avocado, cubed into bite-sized pieces
½	piece, small	red bell pepper, cored, deseeded, julienned
½	head, small	purple cabbage, cored, shredded
½	head, small	green or white cabbage, cored, shredded
12	stalks	chives, minced

For dressing

½	cup	peanut butter, organic
3	Tbsp.	hot or freshly boiled water, add more if needed
2	Tbsp.	rice wine vinegar

2	Tbsp.	*stevia*
2	tsp.	sea or kosher salt
¼	tsp.	sesame oil
1	piece, small	lime, freshly juiced

You will also need:

1	piece, small	mixing bowl
1	piece, large	salad bowl

Directions:

1. <u>To make dressing</u>: combine all ingredients in a small mixing bowl. Whisk well.

2. <u>To make salad</u>: combine all ingredients into large salad bowl. Drizzle 2 tablespoon of dressings on top. Toss salad well to combine. Divide into 4 equal portions.

3. <u>To serve</u>: plate one portion of salad on plate. Drizzle more dressing, if desired. Serve immediately.

Recipe #22: Beef Stroganoff with Zucchini Pasta
Yields 4 servings, recommended serving size: 1½ cup per meal

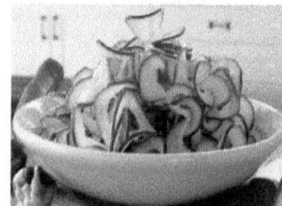

Ingredients:

2	piece, large	zucchini, processed into flat noodles using *spiralizer*, or shaved thin using vegetable peeler, rinsed, drained well, divide into 4 equal portions

For stroganoff

1	pound	ground beef, 90% lean
1	clove, large	garlic, minced
1	piece, large	white onion, minced
1	Tbsp.	almond flour
1	Tbsp.	olive oil
1	tsp.	**Homemade Butter**
1	cup	**Homemade Beef Broth**
½	cup	sour cream
-	-	salt, to taste
-	-	white pepper, to taste
-	pinch	red pepper flakes

You will also need:

-	-	large non-stick saucepan

Directions:

1. Melt butter in skillet set over medium heat. Add in ground beef. Brown meat while breaking up larger clumps. Remove beef from pan.
2. Pour oil in same skillet. Sauté onion and garlic until former is limp and transparent.
3. Add in almond flour. Stir until flour clumps together. Carefully pour in beef broth. Stir until most of flour dissolves.
4. Except for sour cream, stir in remaining ingredients, including partially cooked ground beef. Taste. Adjust seasoning if needed. Put lid on. Turn down heat to lowest setting. Let stroganoff cook for 10 to 12 minutes.
5. Turn off heat. Add in sour cream just before serving. Divide into 4 portions. Allow to cool slightly so as not to overcook zucchini noodles.

6. To serve: plate zucchini noodles. Top off with 1 portion of stroganoff. Serve.

Recipe #23: Beef and Mushroom Stroganoff with Zucchini Pasta
Yields 4 servings, recommended serving size: 1½ cup per meal

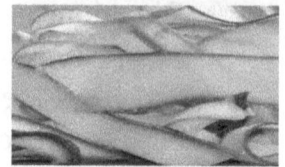

Ingredients:

| 2 | piece, large | zucchini, processed into flat noodles using *spiralizer*, or shaved thin using vegetable peeler, rinsed, drained well, divide into 4 equal portions |

For the beef

1	pound	beef tenderloin tips, thinly-sliced (you can ask your butcher to do this for you)
1	Tbsp., heaping	whole wheat flour, finely milled
2	Tbsp.	olive oil
1	tsp.	sea or kosher salt
¼	tsp.	black pepper, add more if desired

For the mushroom sauce

1	can, 15 oz.	button mushroom, pieces and stems, rinsed, drained well
1	clove, large	garlic, minced
1	piece, large	white onion, minced
1	Tbsp.	**Homemade Butter**
1	cup	**Homemade Beef Broth** or **Homemade Mushroom Broth**

½	cup	table cream
-	-	salt, to taste
-	-	white pepper, to taste

Garnish

½	cup	freshly grated *Parmigiano-Reggiano* or any hard cheese of choice, divided into 4 equal portions

You will also need:

-	-	large saucepan or deep wok

Directions:

1. <u>To prepare beef</u>: season tenderloin tips with salt, pepper and whole wheat flour. Massage beef with your fingers until ingredients are well incorporated.
2. Pour olive oil in a large saucepan set over medium heat.
3. Fry tenderloin tips in batches, browning all sides, about 3 minutes. Transfer partially cooked meat to a plate. Set aside.

4. <u>To prepare mushroom sauce</u>: in same saucepan, melt butter in skillet set over medium heat. Sauté onion and garlic until former is limp and transparent.
5. Except for cream, add in remaining ingredients of mushroom sauce, including partially cooked tenderloin tips. Taste. Adjust seasoning if needed. Put lid on. Turn down heat to lowest setting. Let stroganoff cook for 10 to 12 minutes.
6. Turn off heat. Add in cream just before serving. Divide into 4 portions. Allow to cool slightly so as not to overcook zucchini noodles.

7. <u>To serve</u>: plate zucchini noodles. Top off with 1 portion of stroganoff.
8. Garnish with 1 portion of cheese. Serve.

Recipe #24: Quick Fry Chicken with Cauliflower and Water Chestnuts on Wild Rice

Yields 6 servings, recommended serving size: 1½ cup per meal

Ingredients:

| 1½ | cups | uncooked wild or brown rice, cooked according to package instructions, fluff grains using fork, divide into 6 equal portions |

For the quick fry

2	Tbsp.	peanut oil
1	can, 5 oz.	water chestnuts, rinsed, drained well, quartered
1	head, small	cauliflower, cut into bite-sized florets
1	clove, large	garlic, minced
1	piece, thumb-sized	ginger, grated
1	piece, small	red bell pepper, cored, deseeded, julienned
2	stalks, large	leeks, use white parts only, minced (reserve the rest for garnish later)
1½	pounds	chicken thigh fillets, skins removed, diced
¾	cups	**Homemade Chicken Broth**

Seasonings

-	-	salt, to taste
-	-	black pepper, to taste
1	tsp.	*stevia*
1	Tbsp.	fish sauce
½	Tbsp.	cornstarch, dissolved in
4	Tbsp.	water

Garnish:

-	-	leeks, use leftover green parts, minced
1	piece, large	lime, cut into 6 wedges

You will also need:

-	-	large wok or saucepan, preferably non-stick

Directions:

1. <u>To make quick fry</u>: pour peanut oil in wok set over medium heat. Swirl pan around to coat cooking surface evenly.
2. Sauté garlic, leeks, and ginger until aromatic, about 1 minute.
3. Add in diced chicken. Stir-fry to ensure that meat doesn't stick to the wok. Chicken is done when most is seared and golden brown.
4. Add in remaining ingredients. Cook for 2 minutes while stirring often. Turn down heat. Put lid on. Cook for another 15 minutes.
5. After 15 minutes, add in seasonings. Wait for juice to thicken a little, about 1 minute. Stir-fry, then turn off heat. Divide into 6 equal portions.

6. <u>To assemble</u>: place 1 portion of cooked wild rice on 1 side of the plate.
7. Ladle 1 portion of quick fry on the other. Garnish with minced leeks.
8. Squeeze wedge of lime over quick fry. Serve immediately.

Recipe #25: Baked Salmon Fillets with Kale Chips
Yields 2 servings, recommended serving size: 1 fish fillet and 2 cups kale chips per meal

Ingredients:

For the kale chips

1	pound	fresh kale leaves, stems removed, leaves snipped into manageable squares, rinsed well, spun dry
2	Tbsp.	olive oil, add more only if needed
-	dash	coarse or sea salt

For the salmon fillets

2	pieces, 4 oz. each	salmon fillets, choose even cuts or cuts with even thickness
½	cup	sour cream, store bought
¼	cup	**Homemade Cottage Cheese**
¼	cup	*Parmigiano-Reggiano* cheese, freshly grated (substitute Parmesan or cheddar)

Garnish:

-	-	sweet or Spanish paprika
½	piece, small	lemon, cut into wedges

You will also need:

2	pieces, large	baking sheets, lined with silicon mats or parchment paper
-	-	deep baking dish, large enough to fit both salmon fillets, lined also with parchment paper
-	-	cooling racks
-	-	mixing bowls

aluminum foil

Directions:

1. <u>To make kale chips</u>: preheat oven to 350°F or 175°C.
2. Place kale leaves flat on baking sheets.
3. Drizzle oil on top. Season lightly with salt.
4. Bake for 10 to 15 minutes or until kale leaves' edges turn golden or brown.
5. Remove baking sheets from oven. Place on cooling racks. Let kale leaves cool slightly before using.

6. <u>To prepare salmon fillets</u>: combine sour cream and 2 cheeses together in a small bowl.
7. Place salmon fillets on baking dish. Leave space in between.
8. Pour equal portions of cheese mix on top of each fillet.
9. Place baking dish in oven. Bake for 20 to 30 minutes or until cheese on top turns golden.
10. Remove baking dish from oven. Cover with sheet of aluminum foil. Let fillets rest for 5 minutes.

11. <u>To assemble</u>: place a fillet on a plate. Sprinkle a little paprika on top.
12. Spread kale chips around fillet. Garnish dish with a lemon wedge or 2.
13. Squeeze lemon juice on fillet just before eating. Serve.

Recipe #26: Pan-Fried Tuna Steaks with Spicy Cauliflower Pops
Yields 2 servings, recommended serving size: 1 tuna steak and 1 cup cauliflower pops per meal

Ingredients:

For the cauliflower pops

1	head, medium	cauliflower, cut into bite-sized florets, rinsed, drained well
2	Tbsp.	olive oil, add more only if needed
-	dash	coarse or sea salt
-	dash	white pepper
-	dash	curry powder
-	dash	cayenne powder

For the tuna steaks

2	pieces, 8 oz. each	bone-in tuna steaks, skins snipped at the mid-lines to prevent meat from curling
-	pinch	coarse or kosher salt
1	Tbsp.	olive oil

Garnish:

1	Tbsp.	**Homemade Garlic and Parsley Butter**, divided
2	Tbsp.	toasted garlic flakes, divided
½	piece, small	lemon, cut into wedges

You will also need:

2	pieces, large	baking sheets, lined with silicon mats or parchment paper
-	-	cooling racks
-	-	paper bag
-	-	aluminum foil

Directions:

1. <u>To make cauliflower pops</u>: preheat oven to 350°F or 175°C.
2. Except for olive oil, toss all ingredients into paper bag. Seal bag and shake well to season florets.
3. Place these on baking sheets, stem or cut side down. Drizzle oil on top.
4. Bake for 15 to 20 minutes or until cauliflower tops turn golden or brown.
5. Remove baking sheets from oven. Place on cooling racks. Let florets cool slightly before using.

6. <u>To prepare tuna steaks</u>: lightly season tuna steaks with salt.
7. Pour oil into skillet set over medium heat. Wait for skillet to turn slightly smoky before adding in steaks.
8. Fry steaks only until sides are seared golden, about 2 minutes on first side, and 1 minute on other side. Do not overcook. Flip once only.
9. Transfer steaks on a plate. Cover with sheet of aluminum foil. Let steaks rest for 5 minutes.

10. <u>To assemble</u>: place steaks on individual plates.
11. Spread equal portions of **Homemade Garlic and Parsley Butter** on top of each steak.
12. Sprinkle equal portions of toasted garlic flakes on top.
13. Add in equal portions of cauliflower pops on each plate.
14. Serve dish with wedges of lemon each. Squeeze lemon juice just before serving. Serve while warm.

Recipe #27: Steamed Meat Log *(Embutido)*
Yields 6 servings, recommended serving size: 1 meat log

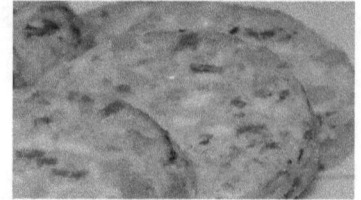

Ingredients:

2	pounds	ground pork, 90% lean
½	link, small	Hungarian sausage, casing removed, ground or minced
2	cups	cheddar cheese, minced
1	cup	raisins
½	cup	**Homemade Pickled Cucumbers**, minced, drained well, seeds removed if any
1	piece, large	carrot, minced
1	piece, small	shallot, minced
¼	piece, small	Tokyo turnip or purple top Milan, minced
¼	piece, small	red or green bell pepper, deseeded, minced
6	stalks	chives, minced
1	Tbsp.	sea or kosher salt
¼	Tbsp.	white ground pepper

You will also need:

-	-	large mixing bowl
6	sheets	aluminum foil
-	-	steamer

Directions:

1. Combine all ingredients in large mixing bowl. Mix very well. Season with salt and pepper. Divide into 6 equal portions.
2. Spoon 1 portion onto a sheet of aluminum foil. Roll into a tight log, sealing the edges well. Roll remaining logs.
3. Steam logs for 45 to 60 minutes. Remove meat logs from steamer. Let cool completely to room temperature before slicing.

4. <u>To serve</u>: remove meat logs from their aluminum wrapping. Slice into thick disks. Plate. Serve while warm, with either ½ cup brown rice or 1 thick slice wholegrain bread.

Recipe #28: Pork Tenderloin Quick Fry
Yields 6 servings, recommended serving size: 1 cup per meal

Ingredients:

2	pieces, small	pork tenderloin, sliced into matchsticks
1	piece, large	white onion, thinly sliced
½	piece, small	red bell pepper, julienned
½	piece, small	green bell pepper, julienned
1	Tbsp.	almond or chestnut flour, finely milled
1	Tbsp.	cooking oil, divided, add more only if needed
1	tsp.	sea or kosher salt
1	tsp.	ground black pepper
½	tsp.	dried pepper flakes (optional)

You will also need:

-	-	large non-stick wok or skillet
-	-	mixing bowl

Directions:

1. Season tenderloin with salt, black pepper, and almond flour. Add in pepper flakes, if using. Set aside.

2. Add ½ tablespoon of oil into wok set over medium heat. Wait for oil to turn slightly smoky before quick frying onions and bell peppers.

3. Stir-fry vegetables only until onions turn slightly transparent, about 1 minute. Remove vegetables from wok immediately. Set aside on a plate.

4. Add remaining oil into wok. Cook seasoned tenderloin in small batches. Stir-fry until golden brown, about 3 to 5 minutes only.

5. Transfer cooked meat into plate. Continue cooking until all meat is done.

6. Return both pork and vegetables in the wok. Toss well to combine.

7. Divide into 6 equal portions. Serve while warm.

Recipe #29: Oatmeal Crusted Chicken Wings and Vegetables
Yields 2 servings, recommended serving size: 2 chicken wings and 2 cups vegetables per meal

Ingredients:

4	pieces, large	chicken wings
6	pieces, large	haricot or green beans, ends and strings removed, sliced into 3-inch long slivers
1	piece, small	aubergine or eggplant, sliced into 3-inch long slivers
1	piece, small	carrot, sliced into 3-inch long slivers
1	piece, small	sweet potato, sliced into 3-inch long slivers
1	tsp.	sea or kosher salt
1	tsp.	ground black pepper
1	tsp.	smoked or Spanish paprika

For the batter

1	cup	almond or chestnut flour, finely milled
1	cup	steel-cut oats
2	pieces, medium	eggs, lightly beaten

		cooking oil, enough to fill fryer ¼ full

You will also need:

-	-	deep fryer or frying pan
3	pieces	bowls
-	sheets	paper towels

Directions:

1. Season chicken wings and vegetables with salt, black pepper, and paprika. Set aside.
2. Preheat deep fryer at medium setting. Add in oil.
3. Place almond flour in a bowl, eggs in another, and steel-cut oats in the last.
4. One by one, dip chicken wings and vegetables in almond flour. Dredge these in eggs, and then coat well in oats.
5. Deep fry chickens first until oats are golden brown on all sides. Do the same for the vegetables.
6. Drain fried pieces on sheets of paper towels before serving. Divide into 2 equal portions.
7. Plate. Serve.

Recipe #30: Apple Cinnamon Lamb Chops

Yields 4 servings, recommended serving size: 1 lamb chop per meal

Ingredients:

For lamb chops

4	pieces, 4 to 5 oz. each	lamb chops, rib-eye, bone in about ¾ inch thick
-	pinch	salt
-	pinch	pepper
-	pinch	Spanish paprika
1	tsp.	**Homemade Plain Butter**
1	tsp.	olive oil

For apple base

2	pieces, large	apples, cored, halved, thinly sliced
1	piece, large	white onion, halved, thinly sliced
-	pinch	cayenne powder
2	Tbsp., packed	brown or unwashed sugar
2	tsp.	cinnamon powder
1	tsp.	olive oil
1	tsp.	butter
½	cup	apple cider vinegar
¼	cup	heavy or double cream

You will also need:

| - | - | non-stick skillet, large |
| - | - | aluminum foil |

Directions:

1. <u>To prepare lamb chops</u>: season meat well with salt, pepper and paprika.
2. Place oil and butter in skillet set over medium heat.
3. Pan-fry lamb chops until seared and golden on both sides, about 5 minutes on the first side and 3 minutes on the other.
4. Transfer meat to a plate and tent with a sheet of aluminum foil. Let lamb chops rest for 3 to 5 minutes.

5. <u>To prepare the apple base</u>: add more oil and butter into skillet.
6. Add in onions and apples. Cook until onions are limp and translucent, about 3 minutes. Stir occasionally and gently, so apples don't crumble.
7. Dissolve cayenne, cinnamon, and brown sugar in apple cider vinegar. Pour mixture into apple base.
8. Return lamb chops to skillet. Spoon apple base on top. Put lid on, and lower heat setting to simmer. Let lamb chops cook for another 10 to 12 minutes.
9. Add in heavy cream. Stir gently.

10. <u>To serve</u>: place lamb chops on 4 individual plates.
11. Divide apple base into 4 equal portions, and ladle these on top of lamb chops.
12. Serve while warm.

Chapter 6: Quick and Health Snack Recipes

* These may also be used as dinner treats.

Recipe #31: Coconut Cream Pie (Almost Instant)
Yields 8 servings, recommended serving size: small slice per meal

Ingredients:

1	piece, 9-inch	pre-baked pie crust, preferably whole-grain or gluten free (this can be bought in specialty or health stores)

For the filling

1	piece, 5 oz.	instant coconut cream pudding mix, or instant vanilla instant pudding mix
2	cups	fresh, tender coconut meat, drained well
1	cup	cold milk
½	cup	cold or chilled coconut milk
½	can, 8 oz.	whipped cream, store-bought

Garnish

½	cups	flaked or desiccated coconut, lightly toasted on dry pan until aromatic and golden
½	can, 8 oz.	whipped cream, store-bought

You will also need:

-	-	large mixing bowl
-	-	rubber spatula

Directions:
1. In a large mixing bowl, combine cold milk, coconut milk, and instant coconut cream pudding mix. Whisk until pudding thickens, about 2 to 3 minutes.

2. Using a rubber spatula, gently fold in whipped cream. Divide mix in 2 equal portions.
3. Spread 1 portion on bottom of baked pie crust. Spread fresh coconut meat on top. Pour in remaining pudding mix. Chill pie well for at least 1 hour.
4. <u>To serve</u>: slice pie into 8 equal portions. Sprinkle toasted flaked coconuts on top. Just before serving, squeeze dollop of whipped cream per slice. Serve immediately.

Recipe #32: Fresh Fruit Salad
Yields 6 servings, recommended serving size: 1¼ cup per meal

Ingredients:

1	piece, large	banana, ripe or overripe, thickly sliced
1½	cup	frozen strawberries, lightly thawed, quartered
1	cup	seedless red grapes
1	cup	seedless green grapes
½	cup	frozen blueberries, lightly thawed
½	cup	frozen blackberries, lightly thawed
½	cup	raisins
1	piece, large	apple, cored, cubed into bite-sized pieces

Garnish

| ½ | can, 8 oz. | whipped cream, store-bought |

You will also need:

| - | - | large mixing bowl |

Directions:

1. In a large mixing bowl, combine all ingredients. Chill well for at least an hour before serving.
2. <u>To serve</u>: ladle recommended portion in small bowls. Squeeze dollop of whipped cream per bowl. Serve immediately.

Recipe #32: Exotic Fresh Fruit Salad
Yields 6 servings, recommended serving size: 1¼ cup per meal

Ingredients:

1	piece, large	banana, ripe or overripe, thickly sliced
2	cups	fresh watermelon, preferably seedless, cubed into bite-sized pieces
1	cup	kiwi fruit, peeled, cubed into bite-sized pieces
1	cup	ripe papaya, seeded, cubed into bite-sized pieces
½	cup	frozen blueberries, lightly thawed
½	cup	raisins

Garnish

¼	cup	raw cashew nuts, freshly toasted on dry pan, cooled completely to room temperature before using

You will also need:

-	-	large mixing bowl

Directions:

1. In a large mixing bowl, combine all ingredients. Chill well for at least an hour before serving.
2. <u>To serve</u>: ladle recommended portion in small bowls. Sprinkle a pinch of cashew nuts per bowl. Serve immediately.

Recipe #33: Creamy Fruit Salad
Yields 6 servings, recommended serving size: 1 cup per meal

Ingredients:

1	piece, large	banana, ripe or overripe, thickly sliced
1	piece, large	apple, cored, cubed into bite-sized pieces
1	can, 15 oz.	fruit cocktail, drained lightly
1	can, 8 oz.	crushed pineapple or pineapple tidbits, drained lightly
1	cup	seedless red grapes
½	cup	frozen blueberries, lightly thawed
½	cup	raisins
2	cups	powdered milk, store bought

You will also need:

| - | - | large mixing bowl |

Directions:

1. In a large mixing bowl, combine all ingredients until powdered milk is well incorporated. Mix gently. Chill well for at least an hour before serving.

2. To serve: ladle recommended portion in small bowls. Serve immediately.

Recipe #34: Sweet Avocado Salad
Yields 4 servings, recommended serving size: 1 cup per meal

Ingredients:

2	pieces, large	ripe avocado, pitted, peeled, cubed into bite-sized pieces
1	can, 12 oz.	evaporated milk, store bought
½	cup	*stevia* or sweetener of choice, add more if desired

You will also need:

| - | - | large mixing bowl |

Directions:

1. In a large mixing bowl, combine all ingredients. Mix gently. Chill well for at least an hour before serving.

2. To serve: ladle recommended portion in small bowls. Serve immediately.

Recipe #35: Assorted Berry Salad
Yields 6 servings, recommended serving size: 1 cup per meal

Ingredients:

2	cups	frozen strawberries, quartered
1	cup	frozen blueberries
1	cup	frozen blackberries
1	cup	frozen raspberries
1	cup	frozen red grapes, preferably seedless, halved
½	cup	*stevia* or sweetener of choice, add more if desired

You will also need:

-	-	large mixing bowl
-	-	muddler or wooden spoon

Directions:

1. In a large mixing bowl, combine all ingredients. Mix gently.
2. Let fruits thaw out at room temperature for 10 to 15 minutes, or until juices render out of the fruits.
3. Using a muddler, gently mash some of the fruits to release more flavor. Mix.
4. Chill again for an hour prior to serving.

5. <u>To serve</u>: ladle recommended portion in small bowls. Serve immediately.

Recipe #36: Watermelon and Lime Ice Lollies
Yields 4 servings, recommended serving size: 1 ice pop per meal

Ingredients:

½	cup	watermelon, cubed, deseeded
½	cup	water
2	Tbsp.	freshly squeezed lemon or lime juice
1	Tbsp.	*stevia* or sweetener of choice, add more if desired

You will also need:

1	square or cube	ice lollies or ice pop container for 4
-	-	blender or food processor

Directions:

1. Process watermelon cubes until smooth. Divide into 4 equal portions and pour into ice pop container, only half full. Freeze until solid, about 1 hour.

2. Combine remaining ingredients. Pour on top of frozen watermelon. Add the ice pop sticks. Freeze again until solid, about 1 hour.

3. To serve: carefully pry out ice lollies. Serve immediately.

Recipe #37: Creamy Banana Slurry
Yields 2 servings, recommended serving size: 1 cup pop per meal

Ingredients:

2	pieces, large	frozen bananas, preferably overripe, roughly chopped
1	cup	frozen yogurt, lightly thawed
¼	cup	ice cubes or crushed ice
1	Tbsp.	powdered milk, store-bought
¼	tsp.	vanilla extract
-	dash	nutmeg powder

Garnish

1	Tbsp., heaping, each	frozen berries of choice

You will also need:

-	-	blender or food processor

Directions:

1. Except for garnish, process all ingredients until smooth.
2. Divide into 2 equal portions. Pour into individual bowls.
3. Top off with chosen berries. Serve immediately.

Chapter 7: Recipes for Homemade Dairy Products

Recipe #38: Homemade Plain Butter
Yields 1 cup of butter, recommended serving size: approximately ½ tsp. per meal

Ingredients:

2	cups	heavy cream, from full fat cow's milk
¼	tsp.	coarse salt (optional)

You will also need:

1	piece	cheesecloth or fine-meshed sieve
-	-	rubber spatula
-	-	blender or food processor
-	-	non-reactive container with lid

Directions:

1. Pour cream into a blender or food processor.
2. Process until liquids and solids separate, about 10 minutes on full power.
3. Using a rubber spatula, scrape out the butter and pour into a cheesecloth or fine-meshed sieve. Squeeze out as much liquid as possible.
4. If using, fold salt gently into the butter. Place in a non-reactive container with a lid. Chill well before using, about 30 minutes.
5. Use as needed.

Recipe #39: Homemade Lemon and Mint Butter
Yields 1¼ cup of butter, recommended serving size: approximately ½ tsp. per meal

Ingredients:

1	cup	homemade butter, preferably salted, at room temperature
1	tsp.	freshly-grated lemon zest
1	tsp.	freshly-squeezed lemon juice
2	leaves, large	fresh mint, finely grated

You will also need:

-	-	rubber spatula
-	-	mixing bowl
-	-	non-reactive container with lid

Directions:

1. Fold all ingredients together in a mixing bowl.
2. Place in a non-reactive container with a lid. Chill well before using, about 30 minutes.
3. Use as needed.

Recipe #40: Homemade Garlic and Parsley Butter
Yields 1¼ cup of butter, recommended serving size: approximately ½ tsp. per meal

Ingredients:

1	cup	homemade butter, preferably salted, at room temperature
1	tsp., heaping	fresh parsley, finely minced
2	cloves, large	garlic, grated

You will also need:

-	-	rubber spatula
-	-	mixing bowl
-	-	non-reactive container with lid

Directions:

1. Fold all ingredients together in a mixing bowl.
2. Place in a non-reactive container with a lid. Chill well before using, about 30 minutes.
3. Use as needed.

Recipe #41: Homemade Cilantro and Lime Butter
Yields 1¼ cup of butter, recommended serving size: approximately ½ tsp. per meal

Ingredients:

1	cup	homemade butter, preferably salted, at room temperature
1	tsp., heaping	fresh cilantro, finely minced
1	tsp., heaping	freshly-grated, lime zest
1	tsp.	freshly-squeezed, lime juice
1	clove, large	garlic, grated
-	dash	black pepper (optional)

You will also need:

-	-	rubber spatula
-	-	mixing bowl
-	-	non-reactive container with lid

Directions:

1. Fold all ingredients together in a mixing bowl.
2. Place in a non-reactive container with a lid. Chill well before using, about 30 minutes.
3. Use as needed.

Recipe #42: Homemade Cream Cheese with Rosemary Butter
Yields 1¼ cup of butter, recommended serving size: approximately ½ tsp. per meal

Ingredients:

1	cup	homemade butter, preferably salted, at room temperature
1	tsp., heaping	cream cheese, at room temperature
1	tsp., heaping	fresh rosemary, minced
1	tsp.	freshly-squeezed, calamondin *(kalamansi)* juice
1	clove, large	garlic, grated

You will also need:

-	-	rubber spatula
-	-	mixing bowl
-	-	non-reactive container with lid

Directions:

1. Fold all ingredients together in a mixing bowl.
2. Place in a non-reactive container with a lid. Chill well before using, about 30 minutes.
3. Use as needed.

Recipe #43: Homemade Spicy Blue Cheese and Chives Butter
Yields 1¼ cup of butter, recommended serving size: approximately ½ tsp. per meal

Ingredients:

1	cup	homemade butter, preferably salted, at room temperature
1	tsp., heaping	blue cheese, mashed, at room temperature
1	tsp., heaping	fresh chives, minced
1	piece, small	bird's eye chili, deseeded, minced

You will also need:

-	-	rubber spatula
-	-	mixing bowl
-	-	non-reactive container with lid

Directions:

1. Fold all ingredients together in a mixing bowl.
2. Place in a non-reactive container with a lid. Chill well before using, about 30 minutes.
3. Use as needed.

Recipe #44: Homemade Garlic, Chives and Tomato Butter
Yields 1¼ cup of butter, recommended serving size: approximately ½ tsp. per meal

Ingredients:

1	cup	homemade butter, preferably salted, at room temperature
1	tsp., heaping	chives, finely minced
1	piece, large	sun-dried tomato, minced
1	clove, large	garlic, minced

You will also need:

-	-	rubber spatula
-	-	mixing bowl
-	-	non-reactive container with lid

Directions:

1. Fold all ingredients together in a mixing bowl.
2. Place in a non-reactive container with a lid. Chill well before using, about 30 minutes.
3. Use as needed.

Recipe #45: Homemade Pizza-Flavored Butter
Yields 1¼ cup of butter, recommended serving size: approximately ½ tsp. per meal

Ingredients:

1	cup	homemade butter, preferably salted, at room temperature
1	tsp., heaping	cheddar cheese, grated
1	tsp., heaping	chives, finely minced
1	piece, large	sun-dried tomato, minced
1	leaf, large	fresh oregano, minced
1	leaf, large	fresh basil, minced
1	clove, large	garlic, minced
-	dash	white powder

You will also need:

-	-	rubber spatula
-	-	mixing bowl
-	-	non-reactive container with lid

Directions:

1. Fold all ingredients together in a mixing bowl.
2. Place in a non-reactive container with a lid. Chill well before using, about 30 minutes. Use as needed.

Recipe #46: Homemade Basil, Cashew and Garlic Butter
Yields 1¼ cup of butter, recommended serving size: approximately ½ tsp. per meal

Ingredients:

1	cup	homemade butter, preferably salted, at room temperature
1	tsp., heaping	raw cashew nuts, freshly roasted, roughly chopped
1	clove, large	garlic, grated
1	leaf, large	fresh basil, minced
-	dash	white powder

You will also need:

-	-	rubber spatula
-	-	mixing bowl
-	-	non-reactive container with lid

Directions:

1. Fold all ingredients together in a mixing bowl.
2. Place in a non-reactive container with a lid. Chill well before using, about 30 minutes. Use as needed.

Recipe #47: Homemade Lemon Buttermilk
Yields 1 cup, recommended serving size: approximately ¼ cup per meal

Ingredients:

| 1 | cup | cow's milk or goat's milk, full fat, preferably chilled for at least 20 minutes |
| 1½ | Tbsp. | freshly squeezed lemon juice |

You will also need:

-	-	whisk
-	-	mixing bowl
-	-	non-reactive container with lid

Directions:

1. Vigorously mix all ingredients together in a mixing bowl. Use long strokes to incorporate as much air into the milk as possible. Buttermilk is done when it thickens a little.
2. Place in a non-reactive container with a lid. Chill well before using, about 30 minutes. Use as needed.

Recipe #48: Homemade Ghee
Yields 2 cups, recommended serving size: approximately ½ tsp. per meal

Ingredients:

1	pound	unsalted cold butter, cubed, preferably homemade, or at least organic and from grass-fed cows

You will also need:

-	-	cheesecloth
-	-	fine-meshed strainer
-	-	saucepan
-	-	spoon
-	-	non-reactive container with lid

Directions:

1. Place butter cubes in a saucepan set over medium heat. Melt completely before turning down heat to lowest setting. Simmer for 10 to 15 minutes. During this time, butter will foam, bubble, subside, and bubble again.
2. Turn off heat when this happens. Cool for 10 minutes before straining.
3. Line a fine-meshed strainer with several layers of cheesecloth. Strain ghee into a non-reactive container with lid. Store at room temperature. Use as needed.

Recipe #49: Homemade Feta Cheese – No Rennet
Yields ¾ to 1 cup, recommended serving size: approximately 1 Tbsp. per meal

Ingredients:

For the cheese:

2	liters	raw cow's milk, full fat
2	liters	raw goat's milk, full fat
3	Tbsp.	freshly-squeezed lemon juice
3	Tbsp.	white vinegar
3	Tbsp.	plain yogurt culture
2	tsp.	coarse salt
-	dash	dried oregano powder
-	dash	dried basil powder

For the brine: (optional)

2	cups	whey, taken after cheese mixture is drained
1	cup	coarse salt

You will also need:

-	-	cheesecloth
-	-	fine-meshed strainer
1	piece, 8 liter	heavy-bottomed stock pot
-	-	wooden spoon
-	-	plastic cheese mold with holes in the bottom, or any non-reactive container
-	-	deep, but small saucepan
-	-	sterilized Mason jar or any glass container

Directions:

1. Place cow and goat milk in stock pot set over medium heat. Bring to a gentle boil before turning heat down to lowest setting, stirring often so skin doesn't form on top, and milk doesn't boil over. This should take 20 to 40 minutes.
2. Turn off heat. Cool for 5 minutes before carefully adding in yogurt culture, lemon and vinegar. Stir once.
3. Cover stock pot with aluminum foil. Leave cheese to curdle for 2 hours.
4. Using your wooden spoon, rake through mixture to break up curds and whey. (**Note**: if the cheese hasn't curdled, boil cheese mix until liquids and solids separate.
5. Season with water with salt, powdered garlic and dried basil or oregano powder. Leave undisturbed for the next 12 hours or preferably, overnight.

6. Line fine-meshed strainer with cheesecloth. Pour cheese mixture through strainer. (Reserve whey for brine, if using.)

7. Gather edges of cheesecloth and twist to remove excess moisture. Tie with twine, and hang cheese to dry for 2 to 4 hours.
8. Place cheese-filled cloth into plastic mold. Secure top with a heavy object (e.g. canned soup) that will press down on the cheese more. This will drain out more moisture. Place in cool place for another 24 hours.
9. Cheese, though lightly salted, is done after 24 hours.

10. To season your cheese properly, place whey and salt in a deep but small saucepan. Let this come to a full boil, and then turn off heat. Cool completely to room temperature before using.

11. Remove cheese from cloth. Cube cheese into bite-sized pieces.
12. Place cheese and brine into sterilized Mason jar. Steep cheese cubes into cooled brine for at least 2 days before using.

13. <u>To serve</u>: gently remove cheese cubes from brine. Drain. Serve as needed.

Recipe #50: Homemade Cottage Cheese – No Rennet
Yields 2 cups, recommended serving size: approximately 1 Tbsp. per meal

Ingredients:

For the cheese:

| ½ | gallon (8 cups) | cow's milk, full fat |
| ½ | cup | white vinegar |

For the seasoning:

| ½ | cup | table cream or buttermilk |
| ⅛ | tsp. | coarse salt |

You will also need:

-	-	cheesecloth
-	-	fine-meshed strainer
1	piece, 8 liter	heavy-bottomed stock pot
-	-	wooden spoon
-	-	saran wrap

Directions:

1. Place milk in stock pot set over medium heat. Bring to a gentle boil before turning heat down to lowest setting, stirring often so skin doesn't form on top, and milk doesn't boil over. This should take 20 to 40 minutes.
2. Once milk comes to a soft simmer, carefully adding in vinegar. Stir. Milk should curdle immediately.
3. Put lid on. Leave cheese to curdle for 30 minutes.
4. Line fine-meshed strainer with cheesecloth. Pour cheese mixture through strainer. (Reserve whey for other use.)
5. Rinse cheese curds under cool running water.
6. Gather edges of cheesecloth and twist to remove excess moisture. Press out as much moisture as possible. Remove curd from cheesecloth.

7. Combine seasonings (table cream and salt) in a small bowl.
8. Mix in cheese curd into seasonings. Cover bowl with saran wrap. Refrigerate for at least an hour before using.
9. Mix cottage cheese prior to serving. Serve as needed.

Recipe #51: Homemade Kefir (Beverage)
Yields 1 quart, recommended serving size: approximately ½ cup per meal

Ingredients:

| 1 | Tbsp. | kefir grains |
| 1 | quart | cow's milk, whole fat |

Seasoning:

| 1 | piece, large | vanilla bean, whole, sliced in half lengthwise |

You will also need:

2	pieces	tall, glass jars large enough to contain more than 1 quart of milk, preferably with air-tight lid
-	-	fine-meshed strainer
-	-	wooden spoon

Directions:

1. Place kefir grains into tall glass jars.
2. Pour enough milk to fill the jar almost to the brim. Put lid on. Let milk sit in a cool place for 2 days, stirring occasionally with a wooden spoon. Do not place milk in fridge. Do not shake glass jar, or stir contents with metal spoon.
3. Strain out the kefir limes. Rinse. Drain.
4. Place rinsed and drained kefir grains into a new, clean tall glass.
5. Repeat steps #2 and #3.
6. After second fermentation, add in vanilla bean into glass jar. Let vanilla steep for at least 12 hours inside the fridge before using.

7. <u>To serve</u>: strain out kefir lime and vanilla bean. Serve kefir well-chilled.

Recipe #52: Homemade Yogurt
Yields 4 cups, recommended serving size: approximately ½ cup per meal

Ingredients:

Yogurt:

4	cups	cow's milk, full fat
3	Tbsp.	plain yogurt, preferably unsweetened with live culture (check product label)

Flavors:

1	tsp., **per ½ cup**	fresh fruits of choice

For the icy bath:

6	cups	cold water
1	cup, heaping	ice cubes

You will also need:

-	-	candy thermometer
-	-	deep saucepan with heavy bottom
-	-	sink for the icy bath
-	-	incubator or yogurt maker, but a thermos will do, sterilized and air-dried
-	-	Mason jar or any heat-resistant non-reactive container with airtight lid, sterilized and air-dried

Directions:

1. Pour milk into deep saucepan set over medium heat. Using candy thermometer, wait for milk to reach 180°F or 82°C, stirring occasionally.
2. Turn off heat. Place saucepan on icy bath to cool down between 110°F or 43°C, and 115°F or 46°C.
3. **Gently** fold in plain yogurt. Pour yogurt into sterilized incubator.
4. Let milk ferment undisturbed for the next 5 hours in a warm place, away from direct sunlight.
5. Refrigerate for 2 hours after fermentation.
6. Stir chosen flavor only when about to serve. Serve as needed.

Recipe #53: Homemade Greek Yogurt
Yields 2 cups, recommended serving size: approximately ¼ cup per meal

Ingredients:

Yogurt:

4	cups	cow's milk, full fat
3	Tbsp.	plain yogurt, preferably unsweetened with live culture (check product label)

Flavors: (choose 1, or a combination of any 2)

-	drizzle, **per ¼ cup**	extra virgin olive oil or any strong-flavored oil (e.g. avocado oil, flaxseed oil, macadamia oil, etc.)
-	dash, **per ¼ cup**	dried or fresh herbs, minced
-	pinch, **per ¼ cup**	coarse salt or powdered spices (e.g. onion powder, garlic powder, powdered paprika, etc.)

For the icy bath:

6	cups	cold water
1	cup, heaping	ice cubes

You will also need:

- | - | candy thermometer
- | - | deep saucepan with heavy bottom
- | - | sink for the icy bath
- | - | incubator or yogurt maker, but a thermos will do, sterilized and air-dried
- | - | Mason jar or any heat-resistant non-reactive container with airtight lid, sterilized and air-dried
- | - | cheesecloth
- | - | colander with glass bowl underneath to catch the whey

Directions:

1. Pour milk into deep saucepan set over medium heat. Using candy thermometer, wait for milk to reach 180°F or 82°C, stirring occasionally.
2. Turn off heat. Place saucepan on icy bath to cool down between 110°F or 43°C, and 115°F or 46°C.
3. **Gently** fold in plain yogurt. Pour yogurt into sterilized incubator.
4. Let milk ferment undisturbed for the next 5 hours in a warm place, away from direct sunlight.
5. Drape cheesecloth over colander with the glass bowl.
6. Strain fermented milk. Gather edges of cheesecloth and twist. Let yogurt drain in the fridge for at least an hour, but overnight is preferable.

7. <u>To serve</u>: spoon out recommended portion in a small bowl. Season lightly with chosen flavors. Serve immediately.
Or
8. Serve Greek yogurt without additional flavors for other dishes.

Chapter 8: Recipes for Homemade Condiments

Recipe #54: Homemade Catsup
Yields 1 pint, recommended serving size: approximately ½ tsp. per meal

Ingredients:

3	lbs., large	fresh, ripe tomatoes, quartered, deseeded
½	cup	apple cider vinegar, preferably sugar-free, and preservative-free
1	Tbsp.	stevia
½	tsp.	coarse salt
1	clove, large	garlic
1	piece, small	dried bay leaf, whole
1	piece	clove
½	piece, medium	shallot, roughly chopped
-	pinch	all spice powder
-	pinch	black, whole peppercorn
-	pinch	celery seeds
-	pinch	red pepper flakes
-	pinch	mustard seeds

You will also need:

-	-	slow cooker or crock pot
-	-	saucepan
-	-	wooden spoon, for mixing
-	-	food processor
-	-	fine-meshed strainer
-	-	non-reactive container

Directions:

1. Place all ingredients in a slow cooker set over medium heat setting. Put the lid on. Set timer for 8 hours. Cook until tomatoes are fork tender.
2. Cool mixture completely to room temperature before removing tomato skins.
3. Discard tomato skins and whole bay leaf. Process the rest in a food processor until almost smooth.
4. Strain the catsup mix while pouring into saucepan.
5. Set saucepan over medium heat. Wait until catsup mixture comes to a boil, and then turn down heat to lowest setting.
6. Simmer until liquid in saucepan is greatly reduced to desired thickness or consistency. Cool completely to room temperature before storing away.
7. Place in a non-reactive container with a lid. Use as needed.

Recipe #55: Homemade Catsup Leather
Yields 1 baking sheet, recommended serving size: 1 2"x 2" square per meal

Ingredients:

½	cup	homemade catsup
-	-	olive oil, for greasing

You will also need:

-	-	offset spatula
1	12" x 17"	baking sheet
-	-	silicon mat, or parchment paper
-	-	cooling rack
-	-	non-reactive container with lid

Directions:

1. Preheat oven to 200°F or 100°C for at least 15 minutes.
2. Line baking sheet with silicon mat, and spray a small amount of oil on top.
3. Spread a thin layer of catsup on baking tray using offset spatula. Make sure surface is almost level, and there are no gaping holes.
4. Bake catsup for 3½ hours to 4 hours, or until catsup is almost solidified in the center.
5. Remove baking sheet from oven immediately. Cool completely before slicing into 2" x 2" squares. Store extra in Ziploc bag at room temperature for up to 7 days. Use leather square as needed.

Recipe #56: Homemade Mayonnaise
Yields 1¼ to 1½ cups, recommended serving size: approximately ¼ tsp. per meal

Ingredients: (Everything must be at room temperature.)

1	piece, large	egg
1	Tbsp.	Dijon or yellow mustard
1½	cups	pure or virgin olive oil (or any mild-flavored oil of choice,) add more if needed
4	tsp.	white wine vinegar or plain white wine
-	-	coarse salt
-	-	white pepper

You will also need:

-	-	food processor with blade attachment (if you are doing this by hand, use a large metal mixing bowl and wire whisk)
-	-	airtight container with lid

Directions:

1. Process egg and mustard in food processor until smooth, about 2 minutes.
2. With machine still running, slowly drizzle in oil in fine, but continuous stream.
3. Do the same for the white wine vinegar.
4. Season with salt and pepper.
5. Store in airtight container. Chill well prior to use. Use as needed.

Chapter 9: Recipes for Homemade Pickles

Recipe #57: Homemade Traditional *Kimchi*
Yields 8 pounds, recommended serving size: approximately ½ cup per meal

Ingredients:

For the cabbage:

| 4 | heads, medium | fresh napa cabbage, root bases trimmed, halved, do not remove core |
| ½ | cup | coarse salt |

For the brine:

2	cups	water
2	Tbsp.	glutinous rice flour
2	Tbsp.	stevia (optional)

Other vegetables:

12	stalks, large	*minari* or Chinese celery, finely minced
8	stalks, large	leeks, finely sliced
8	stalks, large	garlic chives, finely sliced
1	piece, medium	*daikon*, sliced into matchsticks
1	piece, medium	carrot, sliced into matchsticks

Seasonings:

24	cloves, large	garlic, minced
2	tsp.	ginger, minced
1	piece, medium	shallot, minced
2	cups	hot pepper flakes, medium-hot (*gochugaru*)
½	cup	fish sauce

| ¼ | cup | *saujeot* or fermented shrimp in brine, minced (substitute any fermented shrimp product like *Cincalok.*) |

You will also need:

-	-	food-safe gloves
-	-	*kimchi* jar (*onggi,*) or any airtight container with lid
-	-	saucepan
-	-	colander or strainer
-	-	mixing bowl

Directions:

1. <u>To prepare the cabbage</u>: deeply score bases of halved napa cabbages. You want leaves loose but still attached to the core.
2. Rinse cabbages thoroughly. Carefully shake off excess moisture.
3. Sprinkle salt on, around, and in between cabbage leaves – less on the leaves and more on the stems.
4. Let salted cabbages rest for 2 hours, uncovered and at room temperature. Turn cabbages over in 30 minute intervals.
5. Remove thicker part of the cores, but leave a small strip so that leaves are still attached.
6. Rinse cabbages a couple of times. Drain well. Set aside.

7. <u>To make the brine</u>: combine all ingredients in a saucepan set over high heat. Let this come to a full boil. Stir. Turn down heat to lowest setting. Put a lid partially on.
8. Let rice cook for 12 minutes. Stir. Remove from heat immediately. Cool completely to room temperature before using.

9. <u>To make the seasoning</u>: in a large mixing bowl, combine cooled rice with the all the seasonings and the other vegetables. Mix well.

10. <u>To make *kimchi*</u>: spread *kimchi* paste between cabbage leaves. Roll when all leaves are covered. Place these into the *kimchi* jar. Repeat until all leaves are seasoned.

11. Let *kimchi* ferment at room temperature (in a cool, dry place but do not refrigerate) for at least 2 days before using.

12. <u>To serve</u>: get a small amount of *kimchi* from jar. Chop into bite-sized pieces. Serve immediately.

Recipe #58: Homemade Quick Ferment *Kimchi* (Meatless)
Yields 8 cups, recommended serving size: approximately ½ cup per meal

Ingredients:

For the cabbage:

1	heads, large	fresh napa cabbage, cored, shredded
6	stalks, large	leeks, minced
5	cloves, large	garlic, minced
1	piece, thumb-sized	ginger, grated
10	pieces, medium	red radishes, sliced into matchsticks
2	pieces, large	carrots, grated, sliced into matchsticks
1	piece, large	*daikon*, grated, sliced into matchsticks
3	Tbsp.	red chili powder
2	Tbsp.	coarse salt

You will also need:

-	-	food-safe gloves
-	-	*kimchi* jar (*onggi,*) or any airtight container with lid
-	-	large mixing bowl
-	-	colander or strainer

Directions:

1. Combine all ingredients in a large mixing bowl.
2. Using gloves, massage ingredients well, about 2 minutes. This will help vegetables release excess moisture.
3. Repeat previous step in 30 minute intervals for 2 hours.
4. Place *kimchi* in jar, lightly squeezing excess moisture out. Seal. Place jar in a cool, dry place for 1 week to ferment. (Do not place in fridge.)
5. To serve: get a small amount of *kimchi* from jar. Chop into bite-sized pieces. Serve immediately.

Recipe #59: Homemade Pickled Cucumber
Yields 2 pints, recommended serving size: approximately 2 pieces of pickles (½ cup) per meal

Ingredients:

For the pickles:

1½	pounds	pickling cucumbers*, ends trimmed, washed, scrubbed, dried (do not remove skins,) divided
		Note: leave cucumbers whole if small enough, or halved/quartered lengthwise if cucumbers are too thick. Slice into coins, if desired.
4	cloves, large	garlic, peeled, smashed, divided
2	tsp.	dill seeds, divided
½	tsp.	red pepper flakes (optional,) divided
½	tsp.	green or black peppercorns (optional,) divided

For the pickling brine:

1	cup	white vinegar
1	cup	water
1½	Tbsp.	kosher salt

You will also need:

2	pieces, 1 pint each	airtight pint jars with lids, washed well, sterilized, air-dried (make sure jars are heat-

resistant or able to withstand
high heat)
saucepan

\-   \-

Directions:

1. <u>To make the brine</u>: place all ingredients in a saucepan set over high heat. Bring to boil, and then turn off heat immediately. Let brine cool slightly before using.

2. <u>To make the pickles</u>: pack equal amounts of the pickle ingredients between pint jars, adding the prepared cucumbers for last.
3. Pour brine into jars up to ½ inch under brim. Seal.
4. Let pickles cool completely to room temperature before placing in fridge.
5. Let pickles steep for the next 2 days undisturbed before consuming. Unopened bottles can last for up to 1 year in cool temperature. When opened, pickles must be consumed within a week. Use as needed.

* Best cucumbers to use for pickling: Country Fair (do not use in combination with other cucumbers, to prevent bitterness,) Gherkins, Kirby, Muncher (preferably only 4 to 6 inches long,) National Pickling, Persian, Pickling Bush, Regal, and Wallies.

Recipe #60: Homemade Quick Pickled Cucumber
Yields 1 pint, recommended serving size: approximately ½ cup per meal

Ingredients:

For the pickles:

4	pieces, large	cucumbers*, ends trimmed, washed, scrubbed, dried (do not remove skins,) sliced diagonally into thick disks
4	cloves, large	garlic, peeled, smashed, divided
1	tsp.	dried dill leaves
1	piece, large	dried bay leaf, whole

For the pickling brine:

½	cup	white wine vinegar
2	tsp.	stevia
1	tsp.	kosher salt
1	tsp.	mustard seeds
1	clove, large	garlic, peeled, smashed

You will also need:

1	piece, large	airtight pint jar with lid, washed well, sterilized, air-dried (make sure jars are heat-resistant or able to withstand high heat)
-	-	saucepan

Directions:

1. <u>To make the brine</u>: place all ingredients in a saucepan set over high heat. Bring to boil, and then turn off heat immediately. Let brine cool slightly before using.
2. <u>To make the pickles</u>: pack pickle ingredients between jar, adding the prepared cucumbers for last.
3. Pour brine into jar up to ½ inch under brim. Seal.
4. Let pickles cool completely to room temperature before placing in fridge.

5. Let pickles steep for at least 2 hours before consuming. Use as needed.

* Best cucumbers for quick pickling: American cucumbers, Lemon cucumbers, Muncher (preferably longer than 6 inches,) Saladin, Straight Eight, Sumter, Suyo Long, and Tendergreen.

Recipe #61: Homemade Pickled Green Papaya *(Atchara)*
Yields 1 pint, recommended serving size: approximately ½ cup per meal

Ingredients:

Vegetables:

4	pounds	green papaya, julienned
¼	cup	coarse salt
2	pieces, large	carrots, julienned
1	piece, large	white onion, thinly sliced
1	piece, large	red bell pepper, julienned
1	piece, thumb-sized	fresh ginger, julienned
10	cloves, large	garlic, thinly sliced
¼	cup	raisins

For the brine:

2	cups	white vinegar
½	cup	stevia
1½	tsp.	coarse salt

You will also need:

2 to 4	pieces, large	airtight pint jars with lid, washed well, sterilized, air-dried (make sure jars are heat-resistant or able to withstand high heat)
-	-	saucepan
-	-	large mixing bowl, heat-resistant

		colander
-	-	cheesecloth
-	-	saran wrap

Directions:

1. <u>To prepare papaya</u>: place papaya and ¼ cup of salt in mixing bowl. Mix well to combine. Cover bowl with saran wrap. Place bowl in fridge for 24 hours to dehydrate the papaya.
2. After 24 hours, rinse papaya well under running water to remove most of the salt.
3. Place papaya into cheesecloth and squeeze out as much excess moisture as possible.
4. Mix papaya and the rest of the vegetables in a large bowl. Toss well to combine. Set aside.

5. <u>To prepare the brine</u>: pour all ingredients of brine into large saucepan set over high heat. Bring to a boil, and then turn down heat to lowest setting.
6. Simmer until brine is reduced by a quarter. Turn off heat immediately.
7. Let brine cool completely to room temperature before using.

8. <u>To make the pickled papaya</u>: pour brine into the prepared vegetables. Stir gently to combine. Cover bowl with saran wrap. Let vegetables steep for 2 hours in the fridge before bottling.
9. You can consume the *atchara* as is, or bottle these in equal portions in your prepared jars.

Recipe #62: Colorful Pickled Vegetables
Yields 8 to 12 cups, recommended serving size: approximately ½ cup per meal

Ingredients:

Vegetables:

1	head, large	cauliflower, cut into bite-sized florets
1	head, large	broccoli, cut into bite-sized florets
1	piece, large	carrot, sliced into ¼ inch thick coins
6	pieces, large	red chili peppers, whole
4	pieces, tiny	shallots, peeled, trimmed well, whole
1	piece, large	fennel bulb, trimmed well, thickly sliced
½	piece, medium	red bell pepper, cored, deseeded, cut into ½-inch thick strips
½	piece, medium	yellow bell pepper, cored, deseeded, cut into ½-inch thick strips
4	cloves, large	garlic, peeled, whole
¼	piece, small	celeriac root, cut into inch-long strips, halved lengthwise if stalks are too thick
2	Tbsp.	capers in brine, rinsed, drained well
1	tsp.	fennel seeds
-	-	water, enough for boiling vegetables
-	pinch, generous	coarse or sea salt

For the brine:

1	cup	white wine vinegar
1	cup	white vinegar
1	cup	water
½	cup	stevia
1	tsp.	kosher salt
1	tsp.	black or green peppercorns
1	tsp.	Spanish or sweet paprika powder
1	tsp.	white pepper

For the icy bath:

3	cups	cold water
1	cup, heaping	ice cubes

You will also need:

4 to 6	pieces, large	airtight pint jars with lid, washed well, sterilized, air-dried (make sure jars are heat-resistant or able to withstand high heat)
1	piece, large	saucepan
1	piece, large	large mixing bowl
1	piece, large	large bowl for icy bath
-	-	colander
-	-	saran wrap
-	-	slotted spoon

Directions:
1. <u>To prepare vegetables</u>: fill large saucepan ¾ full with tap water. Set pan over high heat. Bring water to a full boil. Add generous pinch of salt.
2. Carefully add in cauliflower flowers. Cook for 6 to 8 minutes, or until vegetable turns one shade darker.
3. Using a slotted spoon, remove cauliflower from boiling water, and dunk florets immediately into icy bath.
4. Do the same for carrots first, then broccoli florets.

5. <u>To prepare the brine</u>: except for stevia, pour all ingredients of brine into large saucepan set over high heat. Bring to a boil, and then turn down heat to lowest setting.
6. Simmer until brine is reduced by a quarter. Turn off heat immediately.
7. Add in stevia. Stir.
8. Let brine cool completely to room temperature before using.
9. <u>To make pickles</u>: drain well cooked vegetables from their icy bath. Transfer to large mixing bowl. Add in remaining uncooked vegetables, herbs, spices and seeds. Toss gently to combine.
10. Pour cooled brine into bowl. Stir gently to combine. Cover bowl with saran wrap. Let vegetables steep for 2 hours in the fridge before consuming or bottling.
11. Pour equal amounts of pickles and brine into prepared jars. Seal. Unopened bottles can last for up to 3 weeks in cool temperature. When opened, pickles must be consumed within 3 days. Use as needed.

Recipe #63: Homemade Traditional Sauerkraut
Yields 4 cups, recommended serving size: approximately ½ cup per meal

Ingredients:

3 to 4	pieces, large	green or white cabbage, damaged outer leaves removed, cored, leaves julienned or thinly sliced, rinsed, drained well
¼	cup	kosher salt

You will also need: (no aluminum/metal cooking instruments or kitchen tools)

1	piece, large	large mixing bowl
1	piece, large	crock pot or any glass or enamel fermenting pot, both pot and airtight lid sterilized well, should be large enough to contain all cabbage slices, packed tight
-	-	saran wrap
1	piece, large	thin towel, for wrapping around the crock pot
1	pair	food grade gloves, optional

Directions:

1. Using clean (or gloved) hands, combine both cabbage leaves and salt in a large mixing bowl. Massage salt well into the vegetables. Cover bowl with saran wrap. Set aside for at least an hour, or until juice comes out of the cabbages.
2. Using clean (or gloved) hands, tightly pack a handful of leaves into a ball, squeezing out excess moisture. (Do not discard.) Place cabbage ball into sterilized crock pot.
3. Repeat previous step until all cabbages are packed.
4. Using your knuckles, pack cabbage leaves more into bottom of crock pot.

5. Pour in cabbage liquid on top. Do not stir. Make sure cabbage leaves are fully submerged under an inch of liquid.

   Note: if there is not enough liquid to fully cover cabbages, create a brine by boiling 1½ tablespoon of kosher salt in 1 quart of water. Cool brine completely to room temperature before pouring. Pour just enough brine to submerge cabbage leaves under an inch of liquid. Discard excess.

6. Securely wrap the mouth of the crock pot with saran wrap. Put the airtight lid on. Wrap entire crock pot with thin towel, and place in a warm place (preferably away from direct sunlight or heat) that will not be moved or disturbed.
7. Allow cabbages to ferment for 4 to 5 weeks.
8. Consume sauerkraut as is, or bottle in sterilized, metal-free, airtight containers.

Recipe #64: Light Beef Broth (Unsalted)
Yields 4 cups or 1 liter, recommended serving size: approximately 1 cup per meal or less

Ingredients:

2	pounds	beef bones, preferably with marrow inside, halved, or cheapest cuts of beef available (ask your butcher to chop beef bones for you, use beef trimmings, if available)
4½	cups	water
1	clove, large	garlic, peeled, whole
1	piece, large	white onion, peeled, whole
1	piece, large	carrot, ends trimmed, roughly chopped
1	piece, large	dried bay leaf
¼	piece, small	celeriac, roughly chopped
1	stalk, large	lemongrass, roots trimmed, roughly chopped
4	stalks, large	leeks, roots trimmed, roughly chopped
4	leaves, large	napa leaves, roughly chopped
1	Tbsp.	black, whole peppercorns

You will also need:

-	-	large crock pot / slow cooker
3 to 4	pieces	airtight container with lid

		colander or strainer
-	-	cheesecloth
-	-	large glass bowl
-	-	saran wrap
-	-	

Directions:

1. Place beef bones in crock pot. Add in the rest of the ingredients. Put the lid on.
2. Set crock pot heat to the lowest setting, and timer to 12 hours.
3. After 12 hours, leave broth undisturbed until it cools completely to room temperature, about 4 to 6 hours.
4. Line colander with cheesecloth. With a large bowl underneath, strain out solids from broth. Discard.
5. Cover bowl with saran wrap. Chill broth in the fridge for at least 6 hours or overnight.
6. Afterwards, remove solidified fat on top. Broth will look gelatinous.
7. Transfer broth to airtight containers. Seal. Reheat and use as needed.

Note: this recipe can also be used for pork broth, using pork bones, pork trimmings, and cheap cuts of pork. The same goes for chicken, veal, and lamb.

Recipe #65: Dark Beef Broth (Unsalted)
Yields 4 cups or 1 liter, recommended serving size: approximately 1 cup per meal or less

Ingredients:

1	pound	cheap cuts of beef with bones, preferably more meat than bones, beef trimmings are okay
1	tsp.	black pepper
1	tsp.	olive oil, add more if needed
4½	cups	water
5	cloves, large	garlic, crushed
2	pieces, large	shallots, roughly chopped
1	piece, large	sweet potato, roughly chopped
1	piece, large	parsnips, roughly chopped
1	piece, large	carrot, roughly chopped
1	piece, large	dried bay leaf
4	stalks, large	leeks, roots trimmed, roughly chopped
¼	piece, small	celeriac root, roughly chopped

You will also need:

-	-	Dutch oven / stock pot / soup pot, large enough to hold all the meat and vegetables
3 to 4	pieces	airtight container with lid
-	-	glass bowl
-	-	saran wrap
-	-	colander or strainer
-	-	cheesecloth

Directions:

1. Season beef cuts with ground pepper. Set aside.
2. Pour olive oil in Dutch oven set over medium heat. Wait for oil to become slightly smoky before browning beef cuts.
3. Brown beef on all sides until golden. Transfer partially cooked meat to a bowl.

4. Sauté shallots and garlic in remaining oil until former is limp and transparent. (Add more oil if there is none left after browning.)

5. Return meat to Dutch oven, and add in the remaining ingredients. Put the lid on. Let broth come to a full boil before turning down the heat to the lowest setting.
6. Simmer broth for 4 hours. Turn off heat, and let broth cool down completely to room temperature, about 2 hours.

7. Fish out the meat. (Reserve for later use for soups and stews.)
8. Line colander with cheesecloth. With a large bowl underneath, strain out remaining solids from broth. Discard.
9. Cover bowl with saran wrap. Chill broth in the fridge for at least 6 hours or overnight.
10. Afterwards, remove solidified fat on top.
11. Transfer broth to airtight containers. Seal. Reheat broth, and use as needed.

Note: this recipe can also be used for pork broth, using pork bones, pork trimmings, and cheap cuts of pork. The same goes for chicken, veal, and lamb.

Recipe #66: Roasted Beef Broth (Salted)
Yields 4 cups or 1 liter, recommended serving size: approximately 1 cup per meal or less

Ingredients:

For the beef:

1	pound	cheap cuts of beef with bones, preferably more meat than bones, beef trimmings are okay
1	tsp.	black pepper
1	tsp.	coarse or sea salt

For the vegetables:

1	Tbsp.	olive oil, for drizzling
2	tsp.	coarse or sea salt
1	head, large	garlic, unpeeled, slice top off
2	pieces, large	shallots, unpeeled, halved
1	piece, large	butternut squash, unpeeled, halved, deseeded
1	piece, large	sweet potato, roughly chopped
1	piece, large	parsnips, roughly chopped
1	piece, large	carrot, roughly chopped
1	piece, large	dried bay leaf
1	sprig, large	fresh rosemary
1	sprig, large	fresh thyme
4	stalks, large	leeks, roots, trimmed, roughly chopped
4½	cups	water

You will also need:

2	pieces, large	baking sheets or trays, enough to hold all the meat on one tray, and the vegetables on the other
-	-	Dutch oven / stock pot / soup pot, large enough to hold all the meat and vegetables
3 to 4	pieces	airtight container with lid
-	-	glass bowl
-	-	saran wrap
-	-	colander or strainer
-	-	cheesecloth

Directions:

1. Preheat oven to 400°F or 200°C. Line baking sheets with parchment paper.
2. Season meat with salt and ground pepper. Arrange these on one baking sheet.

3. Season vegetables with salt. Drizzle with olive oil on cut side.
4. Arrange vegetables cut-side up on the other baking sheet.
5. Place both baking sheets into the oven. Bake for 45 minutes, or until vegetables are fork tender, and beef cuts have crusts.
6. Remove baking sheets from oven. Carefully transfer contents into large Dutch oven.
7. Add in remaining ingredients into Dutch oven set over high heat. Let broth come to a full boil uncovered.
8. Once liquid comes to a boil, turn down heat to lowest setting. Put lid on.
9. Simmer broth for 4 hours. Turn off heat, and let broth cool down completely to room temperature, about 2 hours.

10. Fish out the meat. (Reserve for later use in soups or stews.)
11. Line colander with cheesecloth. With a large bowl underneath, strain out remaining solids from broth. Discard.

12. Cover bowl with saran wrap. Chill broth in the fridge for at least 6 hours or overnight.
13. Afterwards, remove solidified fat on top.
14. Transfer broth to airtight containers. Seal. Reheat broth, and use as needed.

Note: this recipe can also be used for pork broth, using pork bones, pork trimmings, and cheap cuts of pork. The same goes for chicken, veal, and lamb.

Recipe #67: Vegetable Broth (Unsalted)
Yields 4 cups or 1 liter, recommended serving size: approximately 1 cup per meal or less

Ingredients:

1	Tbsp.	olive oil
8	cloves, large	garlic, minced
2	leaves, large	dried bay leaves, whole
2	pieces, large	carrots, roughly chopped
1	piece, large	white onion, roughly chopped
6	stalks, large	leeks, roots trimmed, roughly chopped
¼	piece	celeriac root, roughly chopped
8	sprigs	fresh parsley, roots trimmed, roughly chopped
8	sprigs	fresh thyme, roots trimmed, roughly chopped
4½	cups	water

You will also need:

-	-	Dutch oven / stock pot / soup pot, large enough to hold all the meat and vegetables
3 to 4	pieces	airtight container with lid
-	-	glass bowl
-	-	saran wrap
-	-	colander or strainer
-	-	cheesecloth

Directions:

1. Pour oil into Dutch oven set over high heat.
2. Add in onion and garlic. Sauté until former is limp and transparent, about 1 minute. Take care not to burn garlic.
3. Add in remaining vegetables. Cook for 5 minutes, stirring often.
4. Add in water. Bring this to a boil, uncovered.
5. Once water boils, turn down to lowest heat setting. Put lid on. Cook for 30 minutes or until carrots fall apart when forked.
6. Turn off heat. Let broth cool completely to room temperature, about 30 minutes.

7. Line colander with cheesecloth. With a large bowl underneath, strain out remaining solids from broth. Discard.
8. Cover bowl with saran wrap. Chill broth in the fridge for at least 6 hours or overnight.
9. Afterwards, remove any solidified fat on top.
10. Transfer broth to airtight containers. Seal. Reheat broth, and use as needed.

Recipe #68: Roasted Vegetable Broth (Salted)
Yields 4 cups or 1 liter, recommended serving size: approximately 1 cup per meal or less

Ingredients:

1	Tbsp.	olive oil
1	Tbsp.	coarse or sea salt
1	head, large	garlic, top sliced off
2	pieces, large	white onion, quartered
1	piece, large	carrots, roughly chopped
1	piece, large	sweet potato, roughly chopped
1	piece, small	fennel bulb and fronds, roughly chopped
1	piece, small	egg plant, halved
1	piece, small	squash, halved, deseeded
1	handful	asparagus butts (tough ends)
6	stalks, large	leeks, roots trimmed, roughly chopped
8	sprigs	fresh cilantro, roots trimmed, roughly chopped
8	sprigs	fresh marjoram or basil, roots trimmed, roughly chopped
4½	cups	water

You will also need:

2	pieces	baking sheets, large enough to hold all the vegetables
-	-	Dutch oven / stock pot / soup pot, large enough to hold all vegetables
3 to 4	pieces	airtight container with lid

		glass bowl
-	-	saran wrap
-	-	colander or strainer
-	-	cheesecloth

Directions:

1. Preheat oven to 400°F or 200°C. Line baking sheets with parchment paper.
2. Arrange vegetables on baking sheets, cut side up. Drizzle olive oil on top.
3. Sprinkle salt on cut side surface.
4. Bake vegetables for 30 to 35 minutes, or until squash is fork tender.

5. Season vegetables with salt. Drizzle with olive oil on cut side.
6. Arrange vegetables cut-side up on the other baking sheet.
7. Place both baking sheets into the oven. Bake for 45 minutes, or until vegetables are fork tender, and beef cuts have crusts.
8. Remove baking sheets from oven. Carefully transfer contents into large Dutch oven.

9. Transfer roasted vegetables into Dutch oven set over high heat. Add in water. Let broth come to a full boil uncovered.
10. Once liquid comes to a boil, turn down heat to lowest setting. Put lid on.
11. Simmer broth for 30 hours. Turn off heat, and let broth cool down completely to room temperature, about 30 minutes.

12. Line colander with cheesecloth. With a large bowl underneath, strain out remaining solids from broth. Discard.
13. Cover bowl with saran wrap. Chill broth in the fridge for at least 6 hours or overnight.
14. Afterwards, remove solidified fat on top.
15. Transfer broth to airtight containers and seal. Reheat broth, and use as needed.

Recipe #69: Fish Broth (Unsalted)
Yields 4 cups or 1 liter, recommended serving size: approximately 1 cup per meal or less

Ingredients:

3	pounds	fish heads, collars, tails and bones (you can ask your fishmonger for fleshier pieces, which yield more flavors, do not use cooked fish) Use large chunks of bass, flounder, grouper, halibut or sole. Do not use oily fish like salmon.
1	Tbsp.	olive oil
1	Tbsp.	unsalted butter
2	Tbsp.	black peppercorns
1	handful	fresh parsley, roots removed, roughly chopped
¼	piece, small	celeriac root, minced
2	leaves, large	fresh bay leaves
2	pieces, large	white onions, minced
2	pieces, large	carrots, roughly chopped
4½	cups	water
¼	cup	dry white wine

You will also need:

-	-	Dutch oven / stock pot / soup pot, large enough to hold all fish and vegetables
3 to 4	pieces	airtight container with lid

		glass bowl
-	-	saran wrap
-	-	colander or strainer
-	-	cheesecloth

Directions:

1. Pour butter and oil into Dutch oven set over high heat.
2. Add in onion and sauté until limp and transparent, about 1 minute.
3. Add in remaining ingredients. Bring water to a boil, uncovered.
4. Once water boils, turn down to lowest heat setting. Put lid on. Cook for 30 minutes or until fish heads fall apart when forked.
5. Turn off heat. Let broth cool completely to room temperature, about 30 minutes.

6. Line colander with cheesecloth. With a large bowl underneath, strain out remaining solids from broth. Discard.
7. Cover bowl with saran wrap. Chill broth in the fridge for at least 6 hours or overnight.
8. Afterwards, remove any solidified fat on top.
9. Transfer broth to airtight containers and seal. Reheat broth, and use as needed.

Recipe #70: Shrimp Broth (Salted)
Yields 4 cups or 1 liter, recommended serving size: approximately 1 cup per meal or less

Ingredients:

2	pounds	shrimp and/or prawn heads, preferably fresh or raw as these yield more flavors than cooked ones
1	Tbsp.	coarse or sea salt
1	tsp.	white pepper (optional)
4½	cups	water

You will also need:

-	-	mortar and pestle
-	-	Dutch oven / stock pot / soup pot, large enough to hold all the meat and vegetables
3 to 4	pieces	freezer-safe airtight container with lid
-	-	glass bowl
-	-	saran wrap
-	-	colander or strainer
-	-	cheesecloth

Directions:

1. Season shrimp heads with salt and pepper (if using.)
2. Pound these in batches using mortar and pestle. Place in Dutch oven.
3. Add in water. Set Dutch oven over high heat. Let water come to a full boil.
4. Turn down heat. Let broth cook for another 15 minutes.
5. Turn off heat immediately. Let broth cool completely to room temperature.

6. Line colander with cheesecloth. With a large bowl underneath, strain out remaining solids from broth. Discard.
7. Transfer cooled broth to freezer-safe airtight containers and seal. Freeze.
8. Reheat broth, and use as needed.

Note: you can use the same recipe for crab or lobster stock. Use crab shells and lobster shells. Always use fresh. Ask your local fishmonger to reserve the desired amount for you in advance. Always store your shrimp, crab, or lobster stock in the freezer.

Conclusion

Thank you again for purchasing or downloading "***MTHFR, Whole Food Cookbook & Meal Plans***."

I hope this book has given you more knowledge on how to prepare meals that are MTHFR-friendly. There are many benefits to following MTHFR diet including:

- Lessening or preventing future episodes of chronic pain
- Organic or natural weight loss
- More energy, especially in the morning
- More hours of restive sleep, and
- Better resistance to most infectious diseases, to name a few

Though this diet is somewhat restrictive, it is also gluten-free, low in GI, diabetic friendly, and recommended to people with IBS or Irritable Bowel Syndrome.

After trying out the recipes in this book, the next step is to make your own 7-day MTHFR meal plans, by mixing up the recommended dishes, or better yet: creating or recreating your old favorites by substituting healthier ingredients.

Finally, if you enjoyed this book, then I'd like to ask you for a favor: would you be kind enough to leave a 5-star review for this book on Amazon? It'd be greatly appreciated!

Click here to leave a review for this book on Amazon!

Thank you once more, and good luck with your MTHFR diet!

Check Out My Other Books
GreatMedEbooks.com

Want to Connect with Dr. Purser?

For women's information on progesterone, testosterone and more download some awesome FREE reports:

www.drpursergifts4women.com

Sign up TODAY to Get Your FREE Reports!

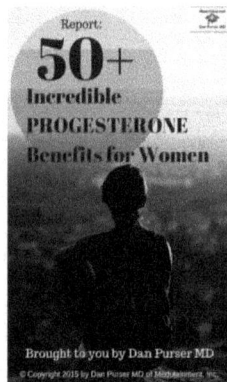

Low levels of progesterone can be treated naturally & optimally in the right situations.

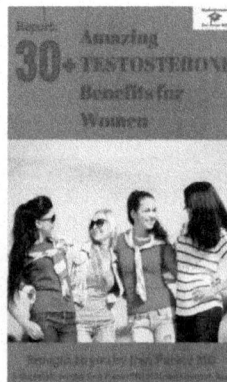

AN AMAZING LIST every woman should own -- all REFERENCED!

NO FOOLING.

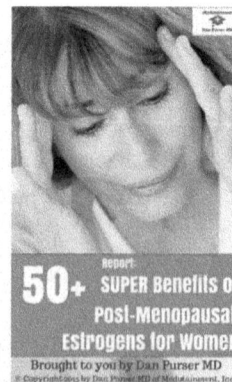

Learn the SUPER BENEFITS of Estrogens in Post-Menopausal Women! This report is fully referenced just for you!

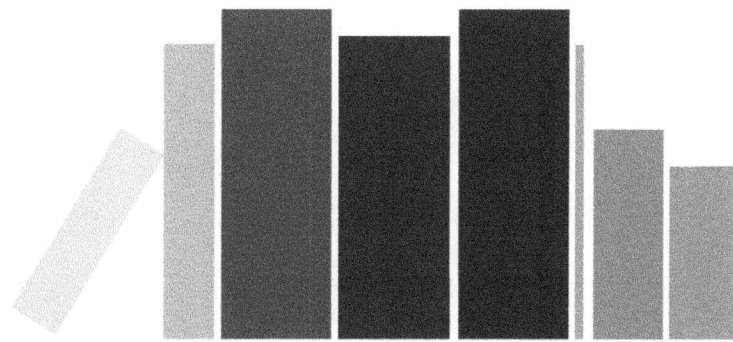

DP PUBLISHING

www.ingramcontent.com/pod-product-compliance
Lightning Source LLC
LaVergne TN
LVHW061259060426
835509LV00013B/1494